Kayla Miriyam Weiner, PhD
Editor

Therapeutic and Legal Issues for Therapists Who Have Survived a Client Suicide: Breaking the Silence

Therapeutic and Legal Issues for Therapists Who Have Survived a Client Suicide: Breaking the Silence has been co-published simultaneously as *Women & Therapy*, Volume 28, Number 1 2005.

Pre-publication REVIEWS, COMMENTARIES, EVALUATIONS . . .

"FINALLY, HERE IS A BOOK THAT SHINES A LIGHT INTO ONE OF PSYCHOTHERAPY'S DARKEST CORNERS: that of a client suicide. Having a client suicide is every therapist's nightmare. This book offers resources, understanding, and most importantly, company for therapists living with or worrying about the nightmare of client suicide. If you have ever lost a client to suicide, read this book for the solace of companionship. If you have been fortunate enough not to have experienced a client suicide, read this book for understanding of an all-too-common event in the practice of therapy. You will be glad you did."

Marcia Hill, EdD
Psychologist in Private Practice;
Author of Diary of a Country Therapist

Therapeutic and Legal Issues for Therapists Who Have Survived a Client Suicide: Breaking the Silence

Therapeutic and Legal Issues for Therapists Who Have Survived a Client Suicide: Breaking the Silence has been co-published simultaneously as *Women & Therapy*, Volume 28, Number 1 2005.

The *Women & Therapy* Monographic "Separates"

Below is a list of "separates," which in serials librarianship means a special issue simultaneously published as a special journal issue or double-issue *and* as a "separate" hardbound monograph. (This is a format which we also call a "DocuSerial.")

"Separates" are published because specialized libraries or professionals may wish to purchase a specific thematic issue by itself in a format which can be separately cataloged and shelved, as opposed to purchasing the journal on an on-going basis. Faculty members may also more easily consider a "separate" for classroom adoption.

"Separates" are carefully classified separately with the major book jobbers so that the journal tie-in can be noted on new book order slips to avoid duplicate purchasing.

You may wish to visit Haworth's website at . . .

http://www.HaworthPress.com

. . . to search our online catalog for complete tables of contents of these separates and related publications.

You may also call 1-800-HAWORTH (outside US/Canada: 607-722-5857), or Fax 1-800-895-0582 (outside US/Canada: 607-771-0012), or e-mail at:

docdelivery@haworthpress.com

---

viewpoints, perspectives, and practices. Each chapter challenges us to move out of the confines of our traditional training and reflect on the importance of spirituality. This book also brings us back to the original meaning of psychology–the study and knowledge of the soul." (Stephanie S. Covington, PhD, LCSW, Co-Director, Institute for Relational Development, La Jolla, California; Author, A Woman's Way Through the Twelve Steps*)*

A New View of Women's Sexual Problems, edited by Ellyn Kaschak, PhD, and Leonore Tiefer, PhD (Vol. 24, No. 1/2, 2001). *"This useful, complex, and valid critique of simplistic notions of women's sexuality will be especially valuable for women's studies and public health courses. An important compilation representing many diverse individuals and groups of women." (Judy Norsigian and Jane Pincus, Co-Founders, Boston Women's Health Collective; Co-Authors,* Our Bodies, Ourselves for the New Century*)*

Intimate Betrayal: Domestic Violence in Lesbian Relationships, edited by Ellyn Kaschak, PhD (Vol. 23, No. 3, 2001). *"A groundbreaking examination of a taboo and complex subject. Both scholarly and down to earth, this superbly edited volume is an indispensable resource for clinicians, researchers, and lesbians caught up in the cycle of domestic violence." (Dr. Marny Hall, Psychotherapist; Author of* The Lesbian Love Companion, *Co-Author of* Queer Blues*)*

The Next Generation: Third Wave Feminist Psychotherapy, edited by Ellyn Kaschak, PhD (Vol. 23, No. 2, 2001). *Discusses the issues young feminists face, focusing on the implications for psychotherapists of the false sense that feminism is no longer necessary.*

Minding the Body: Psychotherapy in Cases of Chronic and Life-Threatening Illness, edited by Ellyn Kaschak, PhD (Vol. 23, No. 1, 2001). *Being diagnosed with cancer, lupus, or fibromyalgia is a traumatic event. All too often, women are told their disease is "all in their heads" and, therefore, both "unreal and insignificant" by a medical profession that dismisses emotions and scorns mental illness. Combining personal narratives and theoretical views of illness,* Minding the Body *offers an alternative approach to the mind-body connection. This book shows the reader how to deal with the painful and difficult emotions that exacerbate illness, while learning the emotional and spiritual lessons illness can teach.*

For Love or Money: The Fee in Feminist Therapy, edited by Marcia Hill, EdD. and Ellyn Kaschak, PhD (Vol. 22, No. 3, 1999). *"Recommended reading for both new and seasoned professionals. . . . An exciting and timely book about 'the last taboo.'. . . " (Carolyn C. Larsen, PhD, Senior Counsellor Emeritus, University of Calgary; Partner, Alberta Psychological Resources Ltd., Calgary, and Co-Editor,* Ethical Decision Making in Therapy: Feminist Perspectives*)*

Beyond the Rule Book: Moral Issues and Dilemmas in the Practice of Psychotherapy, edited by Ellyn Kaschak, PhD, and Marcia Hill, EdD (Vol. 22, No. 2, 1999). *"The authors in this important and timely book tackle the difficult task of working through . . . conflicts, sharing their moral struggles and real life solutions in working with diverse populations and in a variety of clinical settings. . . . Will provide psychotherapists with a thought-provoking source for the stimulating and essential discussion of our own and our profession's moral bases." (Carolyn C. Larsen, PhD, Senior Counsellor Emeritus, University of Calgary, Partner in private practice, Alberta Psychological Resources Ltd., Calgary, and Co-Editor,* Ethical Decision Making in Therapy: Feminist Perspectives*)*

Assault on the Soul: Women in the Former Yugoslavia, edited by Sara Sharratt, PhD, and Ellyn Kaschak, PhD (Vol. 22, No. 1, 1999). *Explores the applications and intersections of feminist therapy, activism and jurisprudence with women and children in the former Yugoslavia.*

Learning from Our Mistakes: Difficulties and Failures in Feminist Therapy, edited by Marcia Hill, EdD, and Esther D. Rothblum, PhD (Vol. 21, No. 3, 1998). *"A courageous and fundamental step in evolving a well-grounded body of theory and of investigating the assumptions that, unexamined, lead us to error." (Teresa Bernardez, MD, Training and Supervising Analyst, The Michigan Psychoanalytic Council)*

Feminist Therapy as a Political Act, edited by Marcia Hill, EdD (Vol. 21, No. 2, 1998). *"A real contribution to the field. . . . A valuable tool for feminist therapists and those who want to learn about feminist therapy." (Florence L. Denmark, PhD, Robert S. Pace, Distinguished Professor of Psychology and Chair, Psychology Department, Pace University, New York, New York)*

Breaking the Rules: Women in Prison and Feminist Therapy, edited by Judy Harden, PhD, and Marcia Hill, EdD (Vol. 20, No. 4 & Vol. 21, No. 1, 1998). *"Fills a long-recognized gap in the psychology of women curricula, demonstrating that feminist theory can be made relevant to the practice of feminism, even in prison." (Suzanne J. Kessler, PhD, Professor of Psychology and Women's Studies, State University of New York at Purchase)*

Children's Rights, Therapists' Responsibilities: Feminist Commentaries, edited by Gail Anderson,
MA, and Marcia Hill, EdD (Vol. 20, No. 2, 1997). *"Addresses specific practice dimensions that
will help therapists organize and resolve conflicts about working with children, adolescents, and
their families in therapy." (Feminist Bookstore News)*

More than a Mirror: How Clients Influence Therapists' Lives, edited by Marcia Hill, EdD (Vol.
20, No. 1, 1997). *"Courageous, insightful, and deeply moving. These pages reveal the scrupulous
self-examination and self-reflection of conscientious therapists at their best. An important
contribution to feminist therapy literature and a book worth reading by therapists and clients
alike." (Rachel Josefowitz Siegal, MSW, retired feminist therapy practitioner; Co-Editor,*
Women Changing Therapy; Jewish Women in Therapy; *and* Celebrating the Lives of Jewish
Women: Patterns in a Feminist Sampler)

Sexualities, edited by Marny Hall, PhD, LCSW (Vol. 19, No. 4, 1997). *"Explores the diverse and
multifaceted nature of female sexuality, covering topics including sadomasochism in the therapy
room, sexual exploitation in cults, and genderbending in cyberspace." (Feminist Bookstore News)*

Couples Therapy: Feminist Perspectives, edited by Marcia Hill, EdD, and Esther D. Rothblum, PhD
(Vol. 19, No. 3, 1996). *Addresses some of the inadequacies, omissions, and assumptions in
traditional couples' therapy to help you face the issues of race, ethnicity, and sexual orientation
in helping couples today.*

A Feminist Clinician's Guide to the Memory Debate, edited by Susan Contratto, PhD, and M.
Janice Gutfreund, PhD (Vol. 19, No. 1, 1996). *"Unites diverse scholars, clinicians, and activists
in an insightful and useful examination of the issues related to recovered memories." (Feminist
Bookstore News)*

Classism and Feminist Therapy: Counting Costs, edited by Marcia Hill, EdD, and Esther D.
Rothblum, PhD (Vol. 18, No. 3/4, 1996). *"Educates, challenges, and questions the influence of
classism on the clinical practice of psychotherapy with women." (Kathleen P. Gates, MA,
Certified Professional Counselor, Center for Psychological Health, Superior, Wisconsin)*

Lesbian Therapists and Their Therapy: From Both Sides of the Couch, edited by Nancy D. Davis,
MD, Ellen Cole, PhD, and Esther D. Rothblum, PhD (Vol. 18, No. 2, 1996). *"Highlights the
power and boundary issues of psychotherapy from perspectives that many readers may have
neither considered nor experienced in their own professional lives." (Psychiatric Services)*

Feminist Foremothers in Women's Studies, Psychology, and Mental Health, edited by Phyllis
Chesler, PhD, Esther D. Rothblum, PhD, and Ellen Cole, PhD (Vol. 17, No. 1/2/3/4, 1995).
*"A must for feminist scholars and teachers . . . These women's personal experiences are poignant
and powerful." (Women's Studies International Forum)*

Women's Spirituality, Women's Lives, edited by Judith Ochshorn, PhD, and Ellen Cole, PhD (Vol. 16, No.
2/3, 1995). *"A delightful and complex book on spirituality and sacredness in women's lives." (Joan
Clingan, MA, Spiritual Psychology, Graduate Advisor, Prescott College Master of Arts Program)*

Psychopharmacology from a Feminist Perspective, edited by Jean A. Hamilton, MD, Margaret
Jensvold, MD, Esther D. Rothblum, PhD, and Ellen Cole, PhD (Vol. 16, No. 1, 1995). *"Challenges
readers to increase their sensitivity and awareness of the role of sex and gender in response to and
acceptance of pharmacologic therapy." (American Journal of Pharmaceutical Education)*

Wilderness Therapy for Women: The Power of Adventure, edited by Ellen Cole, PhD, Esther D.
Rothblum, PhD, and Eve Erdman, MEd, MLS (Vol. 15, No. 3/4, 1994). *"There's an undeniable
excitement in these pages about the thrilling satisfaction of meeting challenges in the physical world,
the world outside our cities that is unfamiliar, uneasy territory for many women. If you're interested at
all in the subject, this book is well worth your time." (Psychology of Women Quarterly)*

Bringing Ethics Alive: Feminist Ethics in Psychotherapy Practice, edited by Nanette K. Gartrell, MD
(Vol. 15, No. 1, 1994). *"Examines the theoretical and practical issues of ethics in feminist therapies.
From the responsibilities of training programs to include social issues ranging from racism to sexism
to practice ethics, this outlines real questions and concerns." (Midwest Book Review)*

Women with Disabilities: Found Voices, edited by Mary Willmuth, PhD, and Lillian Holcomb, PhD
(Vol. 14, No. 3/4, 1994). *"These powerful chapters often jolt the anti-disability consciousness
and force readers to contend with the ways in which disability has been constructed, disguised,
and rendered disgusting by much of society." (Academic Library Book Review)*

Monographs "Separates" list continued at the back

Therapeutic and Legal Issues for Therapists Who Have Survived a Client Suicide: Breaking the Silence

Kayla Miriyam Weiner, PhD
Editor

Therapeutic and Legal Issues for Therapists Who Have Survived a Client Suicide: Breaking the Silence has been co-published simultaneously as *Women & Therapy*, Volume 28, Number 1 2005.

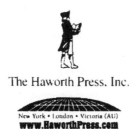

The Haworth Press, Inc.

New York • London • Victoria (AU)
www.HaworthPress.com

Therapeutic and Legal Issues for Therapists Who Have Survived a Client Suicide: Breaking the Silence has been co-published simultaneously as *Women & Therapy*, Volume 28, Number 1 2005.

The development. preparation. and publication of this work has been undertaken with great care. However, the publisher, employees. editors, and agents of The Haworth Press and all imprints of The Haworth Press, Inc., including The Haworth Medical Press® and Pharmaceutical Products Press®. are not responsible for any errors contained herein or for consequences that may ensue from use of materials or information contained in this work. Opinions expressed by the author(s) are not necessarily those of The Haworth Press, Inc. With regard to case studies. identities and circumstances of individuals discussed herein have been changed to protect confidentiality. Any resemblance to actual persons, living or dead, is entirely coincidental.

The Haworth Press. Inc., 10 Alice Street, Binghamton, NY 13904-1580 USA

Cover design by Lora Wiggins

Library of Congress Cataloging-in-Publication Data

Therapeutic and legal issues for therapists who have survived a client suicide : breaking the silence / Kayla Weiner. editor.
    p. cm.
    Includes bibliographical references and index.
    ISBN 0-7890-2376-8 (hard cover : alk. paper) – ISBN 0-7890-2377-6 (soft cover : alk. paper)
    1. Psychotherapist and patient. 2. Psychotherapists–Job stress. 3. Psychotherapists–Legal status, laws, etc. 4. Psychotherapy–Moral and ethical aspects. 5. Suicide victims. I. Weiner, Kayla.
RC451.4.P79T48 2005
616.89′14–dc22
                                           2004012610

Indexing, Abstracting & Website/Internet Coverage

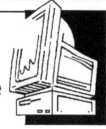

Women & Therapy

This section provides you with a list of major indexing & abstracting services. That is to say, each service began covering this periodical during the year noted in the right column. Most Websites which are listed below have indicated that they will either post, disseminate, compile, archive, cite or alert their own Website users with research-based content from this work. (This list is as current as the copyright date of this publication.)

(continued)

(continued)

(continued)

*Exact start date to come.

(continued)

Special Bibliographic Notes related to special journal issues (separates) and indexing/abstracting:

- indexing/abstracting services in this list will also cover material in any "separate" that is co-published simultaneously with Haworth's special thematic journal issue or DocuSerial. Indexing/abstracting usually covers material at the article/chapter level.
- monographic co-editions are intended for either non-subscribers or libraries which intend to purchase a second copy for their circulating collections.
- monographic co-editions are reported to all jobbers/wholesalers/approval plans. The source journal is listed as the "series" to assist the prevention of duplicate purchasing in the same manner utilized for books-in-series.
- to facilitate user/access services all indexing/abstracting services are encouraged to utilize the co-indexing entry note indicated at the bottom of the first page of each article/chapter/contribution.
- this is intended to assist a library user of any reference tool (whether print, electronic, online, or CD-ROM) to locate the monographic version if the library has purchased this version but not a subscription to the source journal.
- individual articles/chapters in any Haworth publication are also available through the Haworth Document Delivery Service (HDDS).

This volume is dedicated to all therapists who have survived a client suicide
and particularly to those therapists who left the profession
because they did not have adequate support
from colleagues and/or supervisors
to survive this trauma.

ABOUT THE EDITOR

Kayla Miriyam Weiner, PhD, has an independent psychotherapy practice in Seattle, Washington. She received her bachelor's and master's degrees from Temple University and her doctorate in clinical psychology for the Union Institute. Dr. Weiner has written and lectured nationally and internationally on a variety of subjects including but not limited to adoption, morality and therapy, spirituality in the therapy process, political action in the therapy room, anti-Semitism, Jewish women in therapy, and therapist survivors of client suicide. She coedited *Jewish Women Speak Out: Expanding the Boundaries of Psychology* (1995), which received the Distinguished Publication Award from the Association for Women in Psychology in 1996.

Therapeutic and Legal Issues for Therapists Who Have Survived a Client Suicide: Breaking the Silence

CONTENTS

Introduction:
The Professional Is Personal

Kayla Miriyam Weiner

When I got the call that Susan had committed suicide, I refused to believe it. Even after hearing that she had hanged herself in the bedroom, that the police had been there and that the medical examiner had taken her body away, I said, "Are you sure she is really dead?" Once the truth sank in, my next feelings were of panic and fear, followed at various times by confusion, shame, doubt, sadness and relief–to name just a few emotions I experienced.

When I put down the phone I realized I had no idea what to do next. I had been to numerous workshops on suicide prevention and just as many on how to assess for suicidality. No one had ever taught me what to do when (or if) this ghastly event was to occur. And that is the reason for this volume. The pain, confusion and stress I experienced, not just about the suicide, but how to handle the family survivors, the client's records, my practice, my life and myself should not have to be borne by others. This topic has to be discussed openly so that therapists can get the support they need at this very difficult time.

When I learned of the large number of therapists who had experienced a client's suicide, I was astounded that I had never knowingly spoken with a person who had had a client kill her- or himself. The Centers for Disease Control (CDC) (1998) in Atlanta estimates that there are about 30,000 suicides a year in the United States. It is estimated that half of those people were under the care of one mental health provider at the time of, or within 30 days of, the suicide (and many were probably seeing more than one provider), in which case we are talking about 15,000 clinicians a year that have to deal with the trauma of client suicide. When we include the support personnel in agency settings, the number is hard to fathom. It is difficult to imagine anything that directly af-

[Haworth co-indexing entry note]: "Introduction: The Professional Is Personal." Weiner, Kayla Miriyam. Co-published simultaneously in *Women & Therapy* (The Haworth Press, Inc.) Vol. 28, No. 1, 2005, pp. 1-7; and: *Therapeutic and Legal Issues for Therapists Who Have Survived a Client Suicide: Breaking the Silence* (ed: Kayla Miriyam Weiner) The Haworth Press, Inc., 2005, pp. 1-7. Single or multiple copies of this article are available for a fee from The Haworth Document Delivery Service [1-800-HAWORTH, 9:00 a.m. - 5:00 p.m. (EST). E-mail address: docdelivery@haworthpress.com].

http://www.haworthpress.com/web/WT
Digital Object Identifier: 10.1300/J015v28n01_01

fects so many people not being addressed on a national level. This volume is an attempt to encourage educational institutions and mental health centers to talk about this issue, provide training, set protocols and give proper support to the therapists involved.

The goals of this volume are threefold. One is to open the topic for discussion without blame or shame. The second is to provide a place for others to share their feelings and experiences so therapists can know they are not alone with this trauma. The third is to provide resources to help clinicians deal with one (or more) client suicide(s). The volume will offer legal and therapeutic actions for the clinician after the suicide.

The authors who have written about their experiences in this volume come from four countries, work in private and public settings, span most of the mental health professions, and are female and male of varying ages. Most have experienced a client suicide. The works that follow range from poetic to didactic to spiritual. It seems impossible for a therapist to speak or write about her or his experience of surviving a client suicide without describing the event itself, as well as her or his healing and the process of regaining a sense of professional competence. Although a client suicide is a professional event, each author poignantly shows how the personal cannot be separated. Each indicates that the writing of the chapter is part of her or his process of healing from the trauma; the act of writing for publication (or teaching about this issue) is part of an attempt to make the world better for others. This collection addresses the three primary needs of a clinician who survives a client suicide: time to examine one's feelings and heal, someone with whom to discuss the multitude of feelings, and better preparation in training institutions and agency settings.

Healing from the trauma of the suicide of a client is complicated. Whereas the basic grieving process has stages through which one generally moves, dealing with the suicide of a client adds specific issues through which one moves as well. The first is dealing with the immediate responsibilities after the suicide. The next has to do with the therapist's full range of feelings about the client, the suicide and her- or himself. Concomitantly the therapist must deal with the loss of, and hopefully regaining of, a sense of professional competency. Underlying all is the fear of legal action.

REASONS FOR SUICIDE

There are many reasons why a person might commit suicide. A common belief is that suicide is a response to a feeling of hopelessness or despair. It is thought to be an act of giving up or a form of release or, for some, relief. For others, the act of suicide may be an imitation of someone in their family (or family closet) who has used this as a method of coping with life's difficulties. Still others may use it as an extreme cry to be understood: "I want you to know just how badly I feel." People who support the death with dignity movement believe that there are cogent reasons to end one's life. They contend that if one is terminally ill and/or in excruciating, unremitting pain, one may rationally choose to end one's life, especially if one has no emotional or physical support and/or no financial resources. Whatever the reason for the suicide, there are always those left behind to deal with the death and the loss. This is true for a therapist who has a client complete a suicide.

FEELINGS OF THE THERAPIST

The chapters in this volume illustrate how the immediate response of a therapist to a client suicide varies. Described are feelings ranging from shock (even when the client has been suicidal), to disbelief (a need for denial) and fear (of legal implications). Most people report experiencing many feelings at once. After the initial response, a broad range of feelings may follow as well. The literature indicates that as part of dealing with suicide most therapists question their ability as clinicians and often report a sharp loss of confidence (Jones, 1987; Jobes & Maltsberger, 1995).

The authors in this volume discuss their feelings at the time of learning about the suicide(s), shortly after the suicide(s) and well after. They intimately detail their journeys through their experiences. All describe how they attempt to find meaning in what appears to be a meaningless act. While each chapter is personal and unique, the similarities are significant and intriguing.

COLLATERAL ISSUES
WHICH MAY COMPLICATE FEELINGS

Surely there is no good way to learn about a client suicide. Schultz, in this volume, discusses how a person's feelings may differ based upon how she learns about the suicide. Anderson, in her chapter, describes overhearing someone in her clinic speaking about the suicide of her former client. I got a call from a family member. Even with a suicidal client, the suddenness of the news provokes a reaction with each therapist. One can reasonably expect feelings about a previous death or suicide in the life of the therapist to be recalled at this time.

All the authors address how the presence or absence of professional and/or agency support helped them, or failed to help them, through the initial period following the suicide. Support and a venue to talk about the event will lessen the trauma for the clinician (Hendlin et al., 2000). The chapter by Schultz and the one by Spiegelman and Werth provide extensive proposals for what is needed in training institutions and in supervision in agencies to better aid therapists.

There are various characteristics of the client that may have an impact on a therapist's response to the suicide and how they think of the former client. My personal experiences with suicide have elicited very different responses based upon the manner in which the suicide was enacted. A woman who hanged herself in a place that only her child could find her did not elicit much sympathy from me but rather rage for what she had done to her children. Likewise, I felt little for a woman who shot herself in the head in her partner's home. I felt much more compassion for a woman who arranged all of her legal and financial business, wrote a letter to each of her family and friends in which she took full responsibility for her decision, and killed herself so that no one close to her would find the body. Susan, my client, did not take care of any of her financial business and left her partner of many years without resources. My feelings about the suicide were consequently compounded with anger after seeing the added difficulty faced by the person who loved her.

Life experiences of the therapist may have a bearing on an individual therapist's response. In this volume Anderson connects an experience in her life that bound her to her client, and Rycroft notes that the young woman who died was the same age as her daughter. Grad and Michel explore the possible implications of gender as a variable of response to client suicide. My grieving was complicated by the death of another client about the same time. Whereas Susan took her life, Carolyn died due to medical error. Whereas Susan was suicidal and resisted help, Carolyn was life affirming and embraced life. Both were a loss, but my grieving was substantially different for each woman.

COMPOUNDING FACTORS

All the authors in this volume who have experienced a suicide speak about how the attitudes and treatment by those around them influenced how they dealt with the suicide. The response of immediate colleagues and supervisors is often a mirroring of the prevailing attitude within the field of mental health. In general, the mental health profession has been silent about the posttraumatic effect of client suicide on therapists. This silence breeds shame. If a therapist experiences a client suicide and has never heard the issue addressed by other professionals, it is difficult for the therapist to feel she is not alone. The professional silence may also imply to the clinician that she is in some way responsible for the death of the client. Words can be as devastating as silence. All the authors in this volume who have experienced a client suicide discuss the effect of the words of others. Whether spoken or implied, the sense that "if only" the clinician had done or not done something the client would be alive, is often in the air. In an effort to make sense of the self-imposed death, supervisors and other clinicians must help a therapist review a case for understanding, not blame and shame.

RISK FACTORS FOR CLIENT SUICIDE

Chemtob (Chemtob, Bauer, Hamad, Pelowski, & Muraaoka, 1989) noted that clients with organic, mood, and other psychotic disorders were more likely to complete suicide. Many of the people with these disorders are either being seen in mental health agency settings or are in inpatient treatment settings. Chemtob (1989) also noted that the environments most likely to put a therapist at risk for a client suicide include psychiatric hospitals, psychiatric wards of general hospitals and outpatient mental health agencies. Ironically, these are the very places we most frequently send our least experienced clinicians for internships and practica.

Spiegelman and Werth note in their chapter that the importance of dealing with the crisis of suicide for therapists, under discussion for the past 25 years, has yielded little in the way of academic programs for students. Along with Schultz they specifically address the deficit in training of agency supervisors. Since few have been trained to deal with healthy processing of client suicide, the mental health professions seem to be subjecting the most vulnerable clinicians, interns, to the double jeopardy of the risk of having a client suicide and then leaving them to their own resources when it comes to dealing with result of the suicide.

LEGAL SAFEGUARDS FOR THERAPISTS

Feldman, Moritz and Benjamin's chapter addresses legal issues for clinicians. The authors detail ways in which a therapist can minimize the dangers involved in working with suicidal clients. They discuss no-harm contracts, which, as part of the client's file, demonstrate that the therapist has been duly diligent in monitoring for lethality. The authors discuss the importance of assessing for the need for hospitalization, as well as other important practices that help a therapist protect herself from legal judgements.

James in her chapter discusses, with intellect and passion, the development of her method of screening new clients. Those working in private practice would do well to consider their own limits, not only concerning skills or abilities, but in the time and energy required to deal with someone who is actively suicidal. If a client's initial presentation is one of suicide, a therapist must be cognizant of the consequences of engaging with that person before contracting. If a client becomes suicidal while in treatment and requires more than the therapist is able to give, the therapist may do well to find another clinician or agency with resources better able to provide for the client.

Feldman, Moritz and Benjamin in this volume point out why consultation on a regular basis with written documentation is critical. For the individual in private practice, when a client is suicidal, it may be wise to have the client see a number of auxiliary clinicians and participate in collateral treatment. This gives the therapist assistance with treatment and provides support during the therapy process. It also provides corroboration of any efforts taken in the interest of the client. If qualified peer consultation is not available, or if the case is extremely complicated, it is wise to find someone with a higher level credential or expertise in the particular area of concern and pay for supervision. Again, this should be carefully documented. As an added measure, when I have a client in crisis, I have the client write, in longhand, her or his promises and safety plan and have it signed and dated each session. If a legal action should occur, your actions need to be reasonable and prudent, not psychic.

CONFIDENTIALITY

Immediately following the suicide of my client, I was advised by an attorney not to talk to the very people who could have most supported me–my consultation group. He was concerned that if there was a legal challenge and I needed to call any member of the group in a court proceeding to discuss our consultation about the client, each would also be required to report anything I might have said after the suicide as well. At a vulnerable time a therapist may say things that could be taken out of context and used against her or him. The only legally safe way to process the experience in the stages immediately following the suicide is in a position of legally assured confidentiality, and that may mean paying for therapy or paying an attorney. The question of assured confidentiality in agency settings is unclear. Schultz in her chapter and Spiegelman and Werth in theirs give excellent suggestions for developing appropriate supervisory guidelines for helping therapists if there is client suicide.

THERAPEUTIC ISSUES

It may not be wise to speak with the family of the client immediately after the suicide in any detail, except perhaps to express condolences. However, after a time, based on my personal experience, and as Anderson and Rycroft attest in their chapters, contact with the family can be beneficial to all parties. While giving a presentation on the topic of client suicide at an agency, I was advised by the clinical director that, allegedly based on their insurance policy, therapists in that agency were forbidden to attend any service or have any contact with the survivors. That seems unfortunate to me for the healing of both the family and the therapist. Going to the memorial service or funeral may be not only helpful to the therapist emotionally, it may demonstrate caring to the bereaved family. The purpose of any future contact should be not to disclose confidential information about the client but rather to help the survivors grapple with the loss.

During discussions with individuals and from information gained during presentations I have made, I believe the following issues need further attention.

- It is important that collateral personnel in an agency be considered and included in debriefing. They have often had extensive contact with the client and need to examine their feelings.
- A therapist may want time off immediately after the tragedy or may need to continue to work. Some may want time off weeks or months later, when the immediate shock has worn off and they are able to explore the implications of the event. Time off should be available whenever the individual needs it and not when the administration assumes it is needed.
- There may be some states where, for those working in an agency, time off with pay may be available if the suicide ramifications are considered an "on the job injury." Professional associations would do well to lobby for such a benefit.
- Finally, agencies should be sure their insurance policy protects a therapist against an assault on the license of the clinician and not just a suit against the therapist or agency. Although many individual liability insurance companies cover issues dealing with a professional board, that may not be true for agency policies. Again, professional associations should have this goal as part of their mission.

My hope is that this volume will shed a bit of light on the topic of therapist survivors of client suicide and will allow other clinicians to know they are not alone with their trauma. The resources, general, legal and therapeutic, are presented to help clinicians care for themselves and the family of a client who has committed suicide. It is my hope that this volume will prove useful in all these ways to students, teachers and clinicians in the mental health field.

REFERENCES

Centers for Disease Control (1998). National Center for Health Statistics monthly vital statistics report [Online]. 48(11). Available: http://www.cdc.gov/nchs/fastas/suicide.htm

Chemtob, C.M., Bauer, G.B., Hamad, R.S., Pelowski, S.R., & Muroaka, M.Y. (1989). Patient suicide: Occupational hazard for psychologists and psychiatrists. *Professional Psychology: Research and Practice*, 20, 294-300.

Hendlin, H., Lipschitz, A., Maltsberger, J.T., Hans, A.P., & Wynecoop, S. (2000). Therapists' reactions to the suicide of a patient. *American Journal of Psychiatry*, 157(2), 2022-2027.

Jobes, D.A. & Maltsberger, J.T. (1995). The hazards of treating suicidal patients. In M.B. Sussman (Ed.), *A perilous calling: The hazards of psychotherapy practice* (pp. 200-216). NY: Wiley.

Jones, F.A. (1987). Therapists as survivors of client suicide. In E.J. Dunne, J.L. McIntosh, & K. Dunne-Maxim (Eds.), *Suicide and its aftermath* (pp. 126-141). NY: Norton.

Surpassing the Quota:
Multiple Suicides
in a Psychotherapy Practice

Donna M. James

SUMMARY. The author's experience of several patient suicides provides her with an understanding of her own style of working through this professional crisis. Several studies investigate the number of suicides therapists can expect in their careers. The literature on therapists' reactions to patient suicides describes how therapists are affected, and offers models of stages therapists go through in coping. Therapists are likely to feel personally wounded when patients kill themselves, this wounding appearing as guilt, shame, or denial. Several suicides may increase shame. Facing these injuries is part of the healing therapists must undergo to survive and thrive in work with suicidal patients. In spite of similarities in reactions from case to case, each healing is unique. Experiencing several patient suicides may influence therapists to assess their limitations in working with difficult patients. *[Article copies available for a fee from The Haworth Document Delivery Service: 1-800-HAWORTH. E-mail address:*

Donna M. James is a psychodynamic psychotherapist in private practice in Seattle. She is a student at the Fielding Graduate Institute, working on a doctoral dissertation looking at how psychodynamic psychotherapists make sense of their relationships with patients who commit suicide.

Address correspondence to: Donna M. James, 6869 Woodlawn Avenue N.E., Seattle, WA 98115 (E-mail: dmjames@ix.netcom.com).

[Haworth co-indexing entry note]: "Surpassing the Quota: Multiple Suicides in a Psychotherapy Practice." James, Donna M. Co-published simultaneously in *Women & Therapy* (The Haworth Press, Inc.) Vol. 28, No. 1, 2005, pp. 9-24; and: *Therapeutic and Legal Issues for Therapists Who Have Survived a Client Suicide: Breaking the Silence* (ed: Kayla Miriyam Weiner) The Haworth Press, Inc., 2005, pp. 9-24. Single or multiple copies of this article are available for a fee from The Haworth Document Delivery Service [1-800-HAWORTH. 9:00 a.m. - 5:00 p.m. (EST). E-mail address: docdelivery@haworthpress.com].

<docdelivery@haworthpress.com> Website: <http://www.HaworthPress.com>

KEYWORDS. Suicide, occupational stress, psychotherapists, grief

> *. . . I think what will always be with me, too, a fear that it will happen a second time. I lived through it but then oh, God, if it happens again, then that will mean that I'll have more suicides than most people.*
> *I: Is there a magic that you're just supposed to have one?*
> *Yeah, you're only supposed to have one. I've already had my one, thank you.*

The above quote is from an interview with a therapist in Laura Egerton Wert's (1988) dissertation on therapists' reactions to patient suicides. When I agreed to take Mr. Z. into my practice, I had already had two patients suicide, one at a community mental health center where I first started in the profession and one in my private practice. I guessed there was a 50/50 chance Mr. Z. would kill himself. I had to have a brief chat with myself as I sat in my office with this young man. Was I willing to go through that again? If not, I would have to tell him I could not take him on. If I was willing, I had to be prepared to suffer through the self-doubt, second-guessing, grief, and professional angst that I well knew would accompany the worst outcome of this case.

There was something about him I liked. I had already seen him twice, months before. He had come to me through a referral service of which I am a member. He had interviewed two other therapists from that service; I was the last. The morning after his interview with me, he went to his garage, hooked a plastic tube to his exhaust pipe, fit the other end in through the window of his car, and turned on the motor. Something in him had stopped him. He had dragged himself out of there before he lost consciousness. A few days later his aunt brought him back to my office, insisting he tell me this story, and asking me if I would see him.

I made some decisions that were exactly right for his situation. I said that for me to consider working with him the first thing he needed to do was check himself into inpatient drug treatment to free himself from his marijuana habit and alcohol addiction. He would also need to be working with a psychiatrist who would prescribe psychotropic medication for him. He was to get rid of paraphernalia that could be used in an impulsive move to kill himself. After that he could come back and we would reassess treatment options. Three months later, my stipulations completed, here he was in my office, on an antidepressant and a mild dose of an antipsychotic medicine, and still suicidal. He had gone back to the Southwest where he had grown up, gotten drug and alcohol treatment, was working with a psychiatrist there, and was looking for someone to prescribe his medications here in town. His aunt had gotten rid of the plastic tubing. Everything looked good, except that he still wanted to die. I knew unmistakably that he might see to it that he did. He said he wanted to work with me because he thought there was a small chance I could help him.

I did not know that I could help him, but I wanted to, and I decided to take the risk. Almost as an afterthought, it passed through my mind, "Better me than some poor sap of a therapist who's never been through it before." That should have been a personal red flag. In the years since, I have radically revised my criteria for what constitutes a sap. I have also worked with the pride and confusion that drew me to conclude I could handle it better than someone less seasoned, and that I ought to handle it at all.

THERAPISTS AND PATIENT SUICIDES–THE NUMBERS

I have found no research that claims to be an accurate assessment of the number of therapists who have a suicide or multiple suicides in their practices. All of the available statistics come from researchers who get between 20% and 73% response rates to their surveys. Most of them speculate that the statistics they derive from their data provide minimum estimates of the number of people who kill themselves while in treatment.

Chemtob and his colleagues (Chemtob, Bauer, Hamada, Pelowski, & Muraoka, 1989; Chemtob, Hamada, Bauer, Kinney, & Torigoe, 1988a; Chemtob, Hamada, Bauer, Torigoe, & Kinney, 1988b) conducted national surveys of both psychologists and psychiatrists regarding the frequency and impact of patient suicides. The first of their studies (1988a) is a national survey of randomly selected psychiatrists. Of the 259 respondents, 51% had had a patient commit suicide. No differences were noted regarding number of years of practice, or age of the psychiatrist, between those who had experienced patient suicides and those who had not. Among psychiatrists who had had a patient suicide, 55% had been through a second patient suicide. This is about the same probability as having an initial patient kill himself or herself.

In a second study by Chemtob (1988b; 1989) the 51% of psychiatrists from the first study were compared with psychologists' rate of suicide of patients in their practices. Twenty-two percent of responding psychologists reported one or more suicides. The characteristics these researchers found that influence the risk of experiencing such suicides include the following factors. Specialized postdoctoral training reduces the risk of suiciding patients. Female therapists report fewer suicides than male therapists. Psychiatric hospital workers and those working in psychiatric wards of general hospitals or outpatient mental health agencies are more likely to experience suicides of patients. Those who work with organic, affective, substance-abusing, schizophrenic, and other psychotic disordered patients have more patient suicides.

It is worth noting that one difference age does make according to these studies is that the older psychiatrists had lower levels of guilt and social withdrawal than did their younger colleagues. They also had less loss of self-esteem and disruption to friendships. This study indicates that therapists' distress decreases over time. Nonetheless, in Chemtob et al.'s 1988a study, 57% of psychiatrists who had had patients suicide went through a period lasting no more than six months during which they experienced posttraumatic symptoms of clinical magnitude.

Chemtob et al.'s 1989 publication reports a third survey of both psychiatrists and psychologists. This survey produced data indicating that 28% of the psychologists and 62% of the psychiatrists had had patients suicide. Chemtob noted that once therapists had had one patient suicide, the longer they practiced the more likely they were to have a second patient suicide in their practices. The three factors most correlated with having multiple patient suicides in this study were being a psychiatrist, being older, and specializing in the treatment of adults. O'Reilly, Truant, and Donaldson (1990) found that psychiatrists are more likely than psychologists are to experience a second patient suicide. They report finding in their Canadian survey a mean of 0.12 suicides per year of practice per psychiatrist in their respondents. These respondents were 73 psychiatrists with a mean duration of years of clinical practice of 14.9 years. They worked in a variety of settings.

These numbers amount to a mean of 1.7 suicides per psychiatrist responding. This is not, however, how it happens. There was a wide range of rates from 0 to .9 suicides per year of practice. Forty-three percent of these doctors reported no suicides of patients. The rates are not related to years in practice. These researchers surmise that on average, a psychiatrist can expect one patient suicide every 8 years in practice, but some will have none and others will have several. Of the 122 completed suicides covered in this survey, doctors reported 51% of the patients had made previous attempts; 49% of these patients reported suicidal ideations before committing suicide. This means that about half of the completed suicides were by patients who did not report suicidal ideations to their psychiatrists before they killed themselves.

Other surveys of mental health professionals report a similar range of percentages regarding patient suicides. Goodman (1997) surveyed American Psychological Association members. Of these psychologists, 17.8% to 35.6% reported completed patient suicides, the variation in number depending upon whether the patients were still in active therapy or had left treatment. Even therapists whose patients had already stopped therapy before suicidal behaviors occurred were significantly impacted by such behaviors. Howard's (2000) dissertation surveyed people listed in the National Register of Health Service Providers in Psychology. Her respondents reported 24% had had a patient suicide. A verification group of similar respondents reported 39% had experienced patient suicides. An Australian study (Trimble, Jackson, & Harvey, 2000) of psychologists found that 38.9% of respondents had had patients suicide. Menninger (1991) reports 39% among his psychotherapist respondents. McAdams and Foster (2000) report 23.7% of respondents in a survey of counselors. Harris (2001) reports 42.7% among master's and doctoral-level psychotherapy providers in the state of Alaska. Regarding therapists who have had multiple patient suicides, I have found no further statistics.

THE EXPERIENCE OF LOSING PATIENTS TO SUICIDE

I saw Mr. Z. for three weeks, three times a week. We talked about suicide and about his life–his current feelings and thoughts about wanting to die, his plan if and when he ever decided to try it again, the music he would want to listen to before the event. We looked for the symbolism of his method. We explored the aspects of his personality that wanted to stay alive and the ones that wanted to die. He told me about particular incidents and specific days when his suicidal urges were stronger. We found all the reasons he had to live, what he had to look forward to, who wanted him dead, and who was likely to suffer if he died. We discussed his thoughts after one particular AA meeting about making amends. He was still being medicated by the psychiatrist in the Southwest, but was actively looking for a local doctor who would be covered by his insurance when I went on a one-week vacation. I had asked him to meet with a colleague of mine while I was gone, but he had refused to go. We met for an appointment the evening of my first day back in the office. During that week he had found a local psychiatrist who was prescribing his medication. He told me that doctor had agreed to take him off the antipsychotic medicine, as the dose was so low neither of them thought it was making a difference. I did not know if they were right.

There was a lot to catch up on, so I made a note to address this medication change in another session. He was still keeping suicide as an option he said, and doubted that that would change. His aunt called me two days later, the day before our next scheduled appointment. He had been found dead in his car in the garage of his house the morning after our session, a plastic tube attached to the exhaust pipe, the other end pointed into the car window. She said that just the weekend before she had gone with him to get some new athletic shoes and he had been looking forward to a new activity. Had I had any indication from him that he was thinking about doing this again? Indeed, we had ended our last session exploring that part of him that kept him alive.

Articles and books about surviving a suicide (Alexander, 1991; Hauser, 1987; Dunne, McIntosh, & Dunne-Maxim, 1987; Rudestam, 1990) describe survivors' emotional responses to the self-imposed death of someone close. Survivors go through shock, grief that is often tinged with guilt, anger, sadness, sometimes relief, fear of blame from other people, and an abiding need to make sense of what may seem a senseless and wasteful act. Hauser discusses a number of reasons grieving a suicide can be more difficult than grieving other deaths. These reasons include the suddenness of the event, its violent nature, the guilt survivors often experience, the complications suicide poses to normal grief rituals like funerals and religious services, the blame that survivors are apt to project onto one another, and the withdrawal of social support due to judgements about suicide by friends, neighbors, families, and communities.

For the therapist who loses a patient to suicide, there is both a personal response and a professional response. Those publications written specifically about therapists surviving the suicide of a patient (Anderson, 2000; Bissell, 1981; Chemtob et al., 1989; Chemtob et al., 1988a; Chemtob et al., 1988b; Feldman, 1987; Gorkin, 1985; Grad, Zavasnik, & Groleger, 1997; Hammond, 1991; Hendin, Lipschitz, Maltsberger, Haas, & Wynecoop, 2000; Kinsler, 1995; Litman, 1965; O'Reilly et al., 1990; Rubovits, 1993; Tanney, 1995; Wells, 1991; Wert, 1988) describe the responses the therapist can expect to encounter in herself or himself when a patient commits self-murder. In addition to the personal responses that other survivors endure, the therapist often also experiences a sense of failure and injury to her or his sense of professional identity, expectations of negative judgements by colleagues and blame from the friends and family of the suicided patient, doubts about her or his professional competence, and self-questioning about what she or he might have missed as a clinician that now feels like a lethal mistake. A study of therapists in Slovenia (Grad et al., 1997) reports that female therapists subscribe to more feelings of guilt and shame than do male therapists after a patient suicide. One study (Hammond, 1991) indicated that among health care professionals who had experienced both patient suicides and the suicide of a friend, family member, or acquaintance, respondents felt more responsible for the suicides of patients than for those of people in their personal lives.

Other studies (Gralnick, 1993; Kayton & Freed, 1967; Krieger, 1968; Little, 1992; Marshall, 1980) record the kinds of disruptions evidenced in staff members of hospitals and clinics when there is a patient suicide in such an institution. These studies suggest ways in which the professional settings and communities we work in can support therapists working through their grief. When a suicide takes place within a therapeutic community there is often a need for healing among many members of these larger groups.

In reading through the literature on suicide and therapists coping with patient suicides, and in proceeding through my own work, I have looked to see what collective wisdom can be gleaned from the wounding and healing of therapists who have been through this experience a number of times. Bissell (1981) interviewed 11 nurse therapists with a broad range of years of experience and of diverse ages, who worked with suicidal patients. She asked them about their emotional reactions to suicidal casework over time. Her interviews led her to conclude that among these nurses there were common patterns of feeling states through which they progressed in developmental stages leading to greater acceptance of their work with suicidal patients. She named these stages naivete, recognition, responsibility, and individual choice.

In the naïve stage, nurses felt shock, lack of understanding, avoidance, and denial. In the recognition stage, denial disappeared; fear, anxiety, helplessness, and confusion predominated. The responsibility stage included many of the same feelings as the second stage, but as the nurses gained experience in working with suicidal patients, frustration, guilt, and anger arose. Nurses reached the fourth stage when they acknowledged that the choice of suicide was ultimately the patient's responsibility. Factors such as self-awareness, self-confidence, peer support, length of work experience, understanding of mental illness, experiencing completed patient suicides, bias toward saving lives, and ability to communicate all influenced the nurses' progression through these stages. Experience with completed patient suicides is one factor that ushered Bissell's (1981) nurses out of the stage of naivete and into recognition. Their nursing code to save lives heightened the intensity of the stage of responsibility. Bissell (1981), summarizing nurses' moves from the responsibility stage to individual choice, says:

> Finally, after enough postmortems regarding successful (sic) suicides and positive support from administrators, she was able to work through this stage. . . . Progression to the stage of individual choice was enhanced by her continued effort to learn during supervision, formal education, and/or reading existential therapy methods. Through more indepth self analysis possible through personal psychotherapy, she became aware of her excessive guilt, projected anger, and omnipotence. She was able to change these reactions for ones that place responsibility with the client where it in reality lies. She was then able to intervene more objectively yet with sensitivity and caring. (pp. 78-79)

My own experience suggests that naivete dissolves with a first patient suicide. The other three stages still occur after later suicides, sometimes at a more rapid pace than previously, but not always. Every suicide is different. Having already arrived at the fourth stage regarding the first patient to suicide, holding the belief that the patient is responsible for her or his own choices, does not save the therapist from the throes of recognition regarding this second patient's particular life and death. It does not relieve the therapist from fear, anxiety, and confusion. Nor does it absolve the therapist from having to comb through *this* case to assess the work with *this* patient. The process may be the same, but the details and the intensity vary with the particular case.

Wert (1988) in her dissertation on therapists' reactions to patient suicides had 11 therapists who had had patients suicide describe their experience of these events. She saw four major themes emerge in the interviews. The first theme, the presuicide world, consisted of the set of expectations and beliefs therapists held about their ability to help their patients, the patients' willingness to be helped, the willingness of other people in patients' lives to be helpful, and the nature of the therapeutic attachments the dyads had established.

The second theme, the experience of the disruption, explored the emotional impact of the suicides on the therapists. The factors that influenced this array of powerful emotions included the presuicide expectations and beliefs, the method of the suicides, and the reactions of friends and colleagues. The process of resolution is the third theme that emerged from Wert's data. Resolution involved both the challenges to therapists provoked by the suicides and the methods that they used to come to terms with these deaths. The fourth theme was the reaction therapists had to the interview process, often expressed as surprise that describing their experiences so long after the event could elicit so much emotion.

Looking at my own experience through Wert's (1988) lens, I find that with one patient suicide already digested, the presuicide world of every incoming patient is never naïve, to use Bissell's (1981) term. There is a clearer awareness of the patient's resources, internal and environmental. There is a sharper assessment of the patient's desire for life and health. And there is the recognition of an internal resolution, or at least an ongoing debate, within me, regarding the ability of any therapist to keep patients alive. The nature of the dyadic attachment will be what it is as it develops, and it will influence the intensity of the pain with which I will sit, should the patient die by her or his own hand. If another suicide should occur, shock is likely to be more about this particular patient than about suicide generally. Yet exceeding the patient-suicide quota is a shock in itself. Coping with the stigma was, for me, a more serious part of working through the second and third suicides than the first.

Among the flashes of clarity that pierced through the dark time after my third patient suicide was a familiarity with my own way of working through this particular kind of crisis. Following the second and third suicides, I knew what to expect in my own emotional response, what sequence of emotions and thoughts I go through when a patient takes her or his own life. I was able to surrender to grieving in a way that I could not do after the first one, a way that proved useful in making decisions about how to allocate my time and energy to my assorted responsibilities in order to allow myself time to work through my grief and professional reassessment. I knew how to interact with my family regarding my emotional state to reassure them, and to take responsibility for my well-being from their shoulders. The response of clinic staff and my peer support group after my first patient suicide, and the work I had done to establish a professional community for myself in my private practice, gave me experience dealing with suicide within my professional community. With my second and third patient suicides, I knew whom to contact for support, and how to interact with other professionals who had been involved in the care of my patients.

ON SHAME

One evening a couple of months after my young patient asphyxiated himself with poison gas, I went to a committee meeting of a professional organization of which I am a member. Most of us had been on this committee for some time and knew each other well enough to feel some personal safety with each other. Nonetheless, I found it risky to divulge, when asked how I was, the still tender feelings about the suicide and how I was working my way through my reactions. I talked about having had two other suicides earlier in my practice, and how I was still reeling from the effects of this last one. These women had all been working as therapists for years, and had empathy down to an art. They had all thought about what it would be like to experience this kind of loss, and the various ways the loss would be felt. Yet there was a lingering silence as there always is in these moments when I have just told, just enough silence to leave me wishing I had not exposed myself. I should have left them guessing about the tired sadness in my face. It was just enough silence to leave me wondering, as I always do in these circumstances, what they *really* think of me now that they know this truth about me, this truth that in these moment seems to leave all other truths about me in the shadows.

Then Marian said it, right out loud. "So, you've fucked up three times, have you?" There it was, the thing I fear, the secret opinion I know is going through people's minds, the one that inevitably goes through my own, named and sitting right out there among us. An endless three seconds of recognition elapsed before the laughter escaped my throat, and with it, years of subtle tension. People will look for a way to distance themselves from this experience, to keep it from touching their own lives. This is a thought, one thought, that *will* go through people's mind if I tell this story. Hardly anyone will say it to my face. Nobody but Marian with her cut-to-the-chase sense of humor will pack it with all its complex irony and make it funny. And of course, I will tell this story, because it needs to be told and because sometimes I need to tell it.

The mental health field as a whole has swung back and forth, over time, from a tendency to blame the therapist when a patient in treatment suicides (Grad et al., 1997), to a sense of inevitability. Some writers note that in the general population and in the patient population, including hospitalized patients, and in spite of good treatment, a percentage of people will kill themselves (Barraclough, Bunch, Nelson, & Sainsbury, 1974; Cotton, Drake, Whitaker, & Potter, 1983). In the middle of this range of views, suicide specialists work the field. Researchers work to understand why people kill themselves (Everstine, 1998; Lester, 1987). Others try to predict the particular diagnoses and other characteristics of potentially suicidal people (Pallis, Gibbons, & Pierce, 1984; Pokorny, 1983). Those of us who work as therapists are guided in the assessment of our own skills in this area (Bongar, 1992; Neimeyer & Pfeiffer, 1994). And some specialists try to develop the most effective treatment techniques in working with suicidal patients (Hendin, 2000; Leenaars, Maltsberger, & Neimeyer, 1994; Schwartz, Flinn, & Slawson, 1974).

When something goes wrong, and choosing death over life in most cases in Western culture does strike most of us as something gone wrong, we wish to assign blame. We as a profession tend to take on the responsibility for saving people's lives, even those people who crave to be relieved of those lives. We are expected, and expect ourselves, to contain the suicidal patient's anxiety and suffering long enough for her or him to rediscover the desire to live. There is no doubt in my mind that sometimes the work we do contributes to the factors leading up to a patient's death at her or his own hands. We will sometimes not see warning signs. Our blind spots will get in the way of treatment (Modestin, 1987). We will make misguided interventions. Of the 26 therapists in Hendin et al.'s (2000) study of therapists who had experienced a patient suicide, 21 said that in hindsight they would have changed at least one aspect of the patient's treatment. In hindsight, I would have talked that night with Mr. Z. about the change in his medication. I would have explored what it meant to him that he had found a doctor who agreed to take him off an antipsychotic medication that had been working well for months.

We struggle with our personal and professional pride, sometimes looking to absolve ourselves from our patients' decisions. We inevitably wander back and forth between denying our own culpability, assuming the guilt for having failed our suicided patients, blaming someone else for the patient's suffering, and blaming our dead patients for betraying our therapeutic relationships. We come to be the bearers of the pain of failed lives and failed relationships. When we struggle through the grief of a patient's death by suicide, we do double duty, personal and professional.

THE HEALING

The long line of therapists who have experienced patient suicides includes Sigmund Freud, Donald Winnicott, and Ludwig Binswanger, to name a few of the famous. Like Gorkin (1985) and a host of researchers (Bissell, 1981; Hendin et al., 2000; Howard, 2000; Tanney, 1995; Wert, 1988) who have looked at therapists' healing from a patient suicide, I believe that short of being Binswanger in the early years of the twentieth century, with his certainty that existential despair will lead some patients to kill themselves and there is nothing we can do for them (Binswanger, 1958), therapists who have patients who suicide will go through a period of self-questioning. In addition to grieving, we will ask ourselves if, when, and how we may have missed something, where a different intervention might have prevented this tragedy. We will read the books and dive into the articles on suicide assessment and prevention. This part of working through has been an important part of my work in all three cases. The conclusion that we have done the best we could needs to be a conclusion hard-won. We must look in all the corners of the therapy that preceded a suicide to get as close to the truth as possible. Denial will not help; it will, instead, ensconce us deeper in our own pathology. Still, we can never really know what might have been. We are, in most cases, left with ambiguity.

But the guilt, appropriate or not, must eventually be gotten through. Gorkin (1985) succinctly slices it like this: "Two factors affect the therapist's ability to accept this ambiguity and work through the loss: (a) the degree of omnipotence in the therapist's therapeutic strivings, and (b) the nature of the therapist's relationship to the patient" (p. 5). Gorkin sees the first factor, omnipotence, as manifesting either in a sense of worthlessness as a therapist, or as excessive denial of guilt. In both cases, the depressive stance, and the defense against the professional injury, there is an element of fantasized omnipotence. The second factor, the relationship with the patient, involves the extent to which the therapist's attachment to the patient leads to hostility, conscious or otherwise, toward the patient–for the loss, for the betrayal, for the abandonment.

Subscribing to a broader range of human motivations than Gorkin (1985) seems to do, I find his second influencing factor more complicated. There were events and feelings that accompanied the last of my three patient suicides that left me feeling still attached to this gifted young man who had chosen to end his life. This third suicide was both similar to, and different from, the previous two. The intensity of our short time together, and my experience of the profound disconnect at his funeral between his internal world and the world of friends and family among whom he had lived, nagged at me longer and harder than previous experiences had done.

I had taken in his suffering and his longing for connection, and had not been given enough time to sort through it in myself in order to be able to help him find ways to cope in his own life. Beside the anger of the betrayal, there was for me sadness, disappointment, and regret. And there was frustration at not being allowed to do my job. In spite of his death, I felt a need to work through whatever he had left with me that was still unfinished. In a conversation I had with another therapist who has had three patients suicide, this psychologist, 25 years in the field, described to me the greater intensity of his pain after his third and recent patient suicide. This patient had been a successful, intelligent woman with whom he had been engaged in therapy for several years. She had killed herself without a word of warning. The process of working through a patient suicide may be the same in all cases, but some people hurt us more than others do, and the level of our pain depends to some degree on our personal attachment.

Like Gorkin (1985), I believe that some level of personal and/or professional injury on the therapist's part is probable. If the therapist has experienced more than one such loss, all the philosophical resolve achieved in working through the first such incident may well be swept away by a second. After my third patient suicide, I was dubbing myself "Queen o' Death," in my more unhinged and private moments. There are, in such work-throughs, moments spent in the collapse of mental space where there is no room for reflection, and only room for a person's worst suspicions about herself or himself. As the work proceeds, space develops around those psychotic moments, space for thought, ambiguity, complexity, and emotional fullness. Making a space large enough and staying in it long enough for this psychological work to complete itself is the part of the work that allows a person to know the full truth of her or his experience, and hence, allows for the most healing.

FINDING MY OWN LIMITS

As I have become more deeply invested in the notion that therapy's powers lie in its relational nature, I take care what therapy relationships I take on. It is not that I eliminate suicidal patients from my practice. I have most likely helped more people stay alive than I have failed in that attempt. It is not always possible to know who will become suicidal. In fact it is never certain at the beginning of a therapy to what depths of regression the patient will need to sink, to what depressive or psychotic defenses the patient will need to resort, for us to get to her or his whole truth. Yet, at the beginning of a therapy, I now make it as clear as I can that I am only interested in working with people who are interested in getting better. If I am to involve myself deeply with a patient's psychological process, I must insist that that involvement be to some degree on my terms. At this point in my practice, my terms generally include only long-term work if the patient is deeply disturbed.

I recently turned away a woman just out of hospitalization for a suicide attempt. She wanted to see me for the ten sessions her health insurance would cover, but was not willing to go on after that, as her income would not be sufficient to cover my fee. I referred her elsewhere; I would gladly have offered her a reduced fee, but I was not willing to be responsible for convincing her in that ten sessions that her life is worth the price of therapy, even a reduced price. I myself was at one point paying a third of my meager student income for therapy because that is what it took. I have decided to allot myself the right to make a similar requirement for my patients. If I am going to risk spending three to six months devoted in large part to my reaction to a patient's suicide, I expect a commitment from the patient to risk a number of years of coping with her or his own life–and the commitment of the money it takes to do it. This change in my attitude is unmistakably for my own protection, not the patient's. I no longer believe I have the power, or the mandate, to keep people alive, contrary to the majority stance in the profession. Within the contracting process at the beginning of the therapy, I want a new patient to know that we are both on the line, that my engagement is deep, and that my life, at least my professional life, will suffer too.

I would like this not to be the case. I would like to think that after three patient suicides and the development of a strong philosophical belief that my patient is ultimately responsible for her or his own choices, that I can detach easier, recover quicker, grieve faster than I do. But in fact, it takes three to six months of serious psychological work for me to heal from a patient's suicide.

This is so presumably because of my own psychological makeup. Yet this recovery time corresponds to the experience of many other therapists who have been through at least one patient suicide. Three to six months feels like a significant portion of my life to be infused with the details of somebody else's life over which I no longer have any influence whatever. So I limit my practice to minimize the risk to myself. Other therapists have, no doubt, made other decisions for themselves. Some take it upon themselves to research ways to predict and intervene. Some quit practice altogether. Responsible practice necessitates coming to terms with our personal skills and limitations and living with the consequences.

Suicide, like psychopathic violence, psychotic collapse, and some forms of sexual deviance, is at the far fringe of human behavior, a place few of us like to visit. Yet thinking deeply into minds that operate at these extremes teaches us about our range as a species. We are made to see the limits of our capacity for suffering, the lengths to which we can go when cornered, and the depths to which we sometimes plummet when we lose hope. The jagged edges give us an appreciation for what it takes to live and work in the middle ground, as well as empathy for what it is like to cope every day with profound mental pain. The old line comes to mind: It's a dirty job, but somebody has to do it. It is an odd and interesting job therapists take on, sitting with our patients' suffering. When patients call and announce suddenly that they are stopping therapy, often blaming lack of money, we wonder, sometimes for years, what really went wrong in the treatment. We are left holding the loss. When a patient suicides, we are left holding not only the loss, but also some of the patient's suffering. And we are left holding it alone. It is largely among our colleagues that we find the support to bear it. May this collective work extend that support further into our professional community, holding us all as we hold our patients.

REFERENCES

Alexander, V. (1991). *In the wake of suicide: Stories of the people left behind*. San Francisco: Jossey-Bass.

Anderson, E. J. (2000). The personal and professional impact of client suicide on Master's level therapists. *Dissertation Abstracts International. 60*(09). 4873B. (Publication No. AAT 9944663)

Barraclough. B.. Bunch, J.. Nelson. V.. & Sainsbury. P. (1974). A hundred cases of suicide: Clinical aspects. *British Journal of Psychiatry. 125.* 355-373.

Binswanger, L. (1958). The case of Ellen West: An anthropological-clinical study (W. M. Mendel & J. Lyons. Trans.). In R. May. E. Angel, & H. F. Ellenberger (Eds.). *Existence: A new dimension in psychiatry and psychology* (pp. 273-364). New York: Basic Books. (Original work published 1944)

Bissell, B. P. H. (1981). The experience of the nurse therapist working with suicidal cases: A developmental study. *Dissertation Abstracts International, 42*(06), 2307B. (Publication No. AAT 8126678)

Bongar, B. (1992). The ethical issue of competence in working with the suicidal patient. *Ethics and Behavior, 2,* 75-89.

Chemtob, C. M., Bauer, G. B., Hamada, R. S., Pelowski, S. R., & Muraoka, M. Y. (1989). Patient suicide: Occupational hazard for psychologists and psychiatrists. *Professional Psychology: Research and Practice, 20,* 294-300.

Chemtob, C. M., Hamada, R. S., Bauer, G., Kinney, B., & Torigoe, R. Y. (1988a). Patients' suicides: Frequency and impact on psychiatrists. *American Journal of Psychiatry, 145,* 224-228.

Chemtob, C. M., Hamada, R. S., Bauer, G., Torigoe, R. Y., & Kinney, B. (1988b). Patient suicide: Frequency and impact on psychologists. *Professional Psychology: Research and Practice, 19,* 416-420.

Cotton, P. G., Drake, R. E., Whitaker, A., & Potter, J. (1983). Dealing with suicide on a psychiatric inpatient unit. *Hospital and Community Psychiatry, 34,* 55-59.

Dunne, E. J., McIntosh, J. L., & Dunne-Maxim, K. (Eds.) (1987). *Suicide and its aftermath: Understanding and counseling the survivors.* New York: W. W. Norton.

Everstine, L. (1998). *The anatomy of suicide: Silence of the heart.* Springfield, IL: Charles C. Thomas.

Feldman, D. (1987). A social work student's reaction to client suicide. *Social Casework: The Journal of Contemporary Social Work, 68,* 184-187.

Goodman, J. H. (1997). How therapists cope with client suicidal behavior. *Dissertation Abstracts International, 57*(09), 5918B. (Publication No. AAT 9705345)

Gorkin, M. (1985). On the suicide of one's patient. *Bulletin of the Menninger Clinic, 49,* 1-9.

Grad, O. T., Zavasnik, A., & Groleger, U. (1997). Suicide of a patient: Gender differences in bereavement reactions of therapists. *Suicide and Life-Threatening Behavior, 27,* 379-386.

Gralnick, A. (1993). Suicide in the psychiatric hospital. *Child Psychiatry and Human Development, 24,* 3-12.

Hammond, L. K. (1991). Attitudes of selected health professionals toward suicide: Relations to specialty, professional experience, and personal history. *Dissertation Abstracts International, 52*(3-B), 1777. (ISSN: 0419-4217)

Harris, A. H. S. (2001). Incidence of critical events in professional practice: A statewide survey of psychotherapy providers. *Psychological Reports* Special Issue, *88,* 387-397.

Hauser, M. J. (1987). Special aspects of grief after a suicide. In E. J. Dunne, J. L. McIntosh, & K. Dunne-Maxim (Eds.), *Suicide and its aftermath* (pp. 57-70). New York: W. W. Norton.

Hendin, H. (Ed.) (2000). *The clinical science of suicide prevention.* New York: New York Academy of Sciences.

Hendin, H., Lipschitz, A., Maltsberger, J. T., Haas, A. P., & Wynecoop, S. (2000). Therapists' reactions to patients' suicides. *American Journal of Psychiatry, 157,* 2022-2027.

Howard, E. L. (2000). Incidence and impact of client suicide on health service providers in psychology. *Dissertation Abstracts International, 61*(09), 4986B. (Publication No. AAT 9985639)

Kayton, L. & Freed, H. (1967). Effects of a suicide in a psychiatric hospital. *Archives of General Psychiatry, 17,* 187-195.

Kinsler, P. J. (1995). A story for Marcie. *Dissociation: Progress in the Dissociative Disorders, 8,* 100-103.

Krieger, G. (1968). Psychological autopsies of hospital suicides. *Hospital and Community Psychiatry, 19,* 42-221.

Leenaars, A. A., Maltsberger, J. T., & Neimeyer, R. A. (1994). *Treatment of suicidal people.* Philadelphia: Taylor & Francis.

Lester, D. (1997). *Making sense of suicide: An in-depth look at why people kill themselves.* Philadelphia: The Charles Press.

Litman, R. E. (1965). When patients commit suicide. *American Journal of Psychotherapy, 4,* 570-576.

Little, J. D. (1992). Staff response to inpatient and outpatient suicide: What happened and what do we do? *Australian and New Zealand Journal of Psychiatry, 26,* 162-167.

Marshall, K. A. (1980). When a patient commits suicide. *Suicide and Life-Threatening Behavior, 10,* 29-40.

McAdams, C. R. III & Foster, V. A. (2000). Client suicide: Its frequency and impact on counselors. *Journal of Mental Health Counseling, 22,* 107-121.

Menninger, W. W. (1991). Patient suicide and its impact on the psychotherapist. *Bulletin of the Menninger Clinic, 55,* 216-227.

Modestin, J. (1987). Counter transference reaction contributing to completed suicides. *British Journal of Medical Psychology, 60,* 379-385.

Neimeyer, R. A. & Pfeiffer, A. M. (1994). The ten most common errors of suicide interventionists. In A. A. Leenaars, J. T. Maltsberger, & R. A. Neimeyer (Eds.), *Treatment of suicidal people* (pp. 207-224). Philadelphia: Taylor & Francis.

O'Reilly, M. B., Truant, M. D., & Donaldson, B. A. (1990). Psychiatrists' experience of suicide in their patients. *Psychiatric Journal of the University of Ottawa, 15,* 173-176.

Pallis, D. J., Gibbons, J. S., & Pierce, D. W. (1984). Estimating suicide risk among attempted suicides. *British Journal of Psychiatry, 144,* 139-148.

Pokorny, A. D. (1983). Prediction of suicide in psychiatric patients. *Archives of General Psychiatry, 40,* 249-257.

Rubovits, J. S. (1993). Therapists' reactions to client suicide. *Dissertation Abstracts International, 54*(08), 4405B. (Publication No. AAT 9401810)

Rudestam, K. E. (1990). Survivors of suicide: Research and speculations. In D. Lester (Ed.), *Current concepts of suicide* (pp. 203-213). Philadelphia: The Charles Press.

Schwartz, D. A., Flinn, D. E. & Slawson, P. F. (1974). Treatment of the suicidal character. *American Journal of Psychotherapy, 28,* 194-207.

Tanney, B. (1995). After a suicide: A helper's handbook. In B. L. Mishara (Ed.), *The impact of suicide* (pp. 100-120). New York: Springer Publishing Co.

Trimble, L., Jackson, K., & Harvey, D. (2000). Client suicidal behaviour: Impact, interventions, and implications for psychologists. *Australian Psychologist* Special Issue, *35,* 227-232.

Wells, M. L. (1991). Psychotherapists' perceptions of client suicide: A pheno-menological investigation. *Dissertation Abstracts International, 53*(02), 1112B. (Publication No. AAT 9220589)

Wert, Laura Egterton (1988). The experience of the therapist when a patient commits suicide. *Dissertation Abstracts International. 50*(03), 1128B. (Publication No. 8911770)

Who, What, When, Where, How, and Mostly Why?
A Therapist's Grief over the Suicide of a Client

Gail O. Anderson

SUMMARY. The death of a client by suicide was very emotionally destabilizing to this therapist. She worked hard to distance herself personally from the pain at first and at the same time she found herself overfocused on the "psychological autopsy." She had difficulty accepting new clients and wanted to withdraw from a meaningful appointment to a state advisory committee. Only when she was able to identify with the client's pain and realize how that pain touched her own history of loss was she able to grieve productively. She realized that gender was relevant in her identification with the victim and in sorting out each of their histories of loss. *[Article copies available for a fee from The Haworth Document Delivery Service: 1-800-HAWORTH. E-mail address: <docdelivery@haworthpress.com> Website: <http://www.HaworthPress. com> © 2005 by The Haworth Press, Inc. All rights reserved.]*

Gail O. Anderson, MA, works as a therapist for a nonprofit agency, Lutheran Social Service of Minnesota. She has a passion for working with children, teens and their families. She serves on the Minnesota State Advisory Committee subcommittee on children's mental health and coedited a *Women & Therapy* issue on "Children's Rights, Therapists' Responsibilities" with Marcia Hill, EdD.

Address correspondence to: Gail O. Anderson, Lutheran Social Service, P.O. Box 6069, St. Cloud, MN 56302.

[Haworth co-indexing entry note]: "Who, What, When, Where, How, and Mostly Why? A Therapist's Grief over the Suicide of a Client." Anderson, Gail O. Co-published simultaneously in *Women & Therapy* (The Haworth Press, Inc.) Vol. 28, No. 1, 2005, pp. 25-34; and: *Therapeutic and Legal Issues for Therapists Who Have Survived a Client Suicide: Breaking the Silence* (ed: Kayla Miriyam Weiner) The Haworth Press, Inc., 2005, pp. 25-34. Single or multiple copies of this article are available for a fee from The Haworth Document Delivery Service [1-800-HAWORTH, 9:00 a.m. - 5:00 p.m. (EST). E-mail address: docdelivery@haworthpress.com].

Digital Object Identifier: 10.1300/J015v28n01_03

KEYWORDS. Suicide, therapist reaction, feminist, grief, gender

CONTEXT OF THE THERAPEUTIC RELATIONSHIP

Annie was a slight wisp of girl, blue eyes large in her thin face and a slumped posture like many 11-year-old girls who aren't so sure of themselves. She was well defended behind a flippant yet dramatic presentation which both caught my attention and kept me at bay. Almost her first words to me were, "I hate my life."

I had seen Annie for ten sessions, some of those with her family. Sadly, I had had a difficult time connecting with her. This was one of the most troubling aspects of dealing with Annie's suicide three years later, when she hanged herself in her closet three weeks before her 14th birthday. After she died, I learned that she was scheduled to see me again within a couple of weeks.

I take a lot of pride in my 18 years' work in therapy with a variety of individuals, couples and families. My orientation as a feminist therapist helps me to connect with children and adults I recognize as wounded by a society which continues to scar females and males in different ways. I look for power gone awry. Most certainly I see clients in the context of their larger world which holds too much injustice and abuse of power.

I wondered what led this young woman to choose to use her power in such a final way. I pondered what made her so desperate she chose to be violent to herself, to use her own power to stop her breath and life. I questioned if she knew what she was doing or if she simply acted out how she felt. Why did this happen? What could have prevented it?

MY INITIAL REACTION

I was standing in a church satellite office when the call came through from the mother. They wanted a pastor to come by. Their daughter had killed herself. This teenager had been at the church the night before studying for confirmation and had said to her peers that night, "Suicide is wrong. I would never do it."

I was shocked but tucked the rising feelings back inside neatly and went through my workday knowing that I had six hourly sessions to complete and I needed to be available emotionally to those living. I did call my office to ask them to pull the chart, and I requested my clinical supervisor review it.

At the end of the day I returned to feeling and thinking without the filter of interaction with people working hard on their own lives. I had some thoughts that seemed cold. One of those thoughts was that perhaps the lack of connection I felt with this young woman was diagnostic. I surmised that she felt empty no matter how much others around her cared for her. Was she someone who could not receive love or caring? If so, how did she get that way? While I cannot say whether my thoughts were accurate, I now recognize this defense as my way of not allowing my feelings to surface. I was focusing on her rather than on how I was feeling.

Another distancing thought I had was that it was better she would not have children given the degree of her emotional wounds, because surely her inability to connect would hurt them as well. I conveniently thought about her as a subject, even an object, rather than screaming at the top of my lungs "NO!" as I felt like doing. It was still carefully about her, not me.

THE WAKE AND THE FUNERAL AND CONTACT WITH THE FAMILY SURVIVORS

I chose to attend the wake and to approach the family members with my condolences. It was good to see Annie's oldest sister, a 20-year-old woman who had worked in individual therapy with me a couple of times in her adolescent years. I was able to speak with her mother and father and the other three sisters as well.

As the only therapist who came to this small town, I had another reason to attend. I knew I would see others, particularly her peers, who were affected by Annie's death and I wanted to be a part of their experience. I still didn't own that I was also grieving.

The funeral was important and personal. The pastor was very loving in his attitude toward Annie and her family. He had asked me ahead of time if I had any recommendations for what to include. I said, "Tell them that depression kills. If Annie focused on suicide as the only option, no one could have prevented it." He included those thoughts and compared her to the sparrow who falls from the sky, moving God deeply with grief. Meanwhile I wrote on my funeral bulletin, "Am I jaded? I remain untouched by her, she by me." "Did she have reactive attachment disorder? Did she think she would be found? Did she need to express her emotional pain in the only way that was big enough?"

The family remembered me, and Annie's oldest sister said she'd be coming in to see me. I welcomed her because I do care about her and work well with her. I admit I also wanted to know details or clues the family perceived so that I could do a psychological autopsy. I was hoping it would explain exactly what had happened and why the suicide had occurred. Perhaps I was bargaining that if I had had this information I could have prevented the suicide by doing something differently three years earlier. At this point I was beginning to catch on that I was not untouched by Annie's suicide.

PSYCHOLOGICAL AUTOPSY OF A SUICIDE

Information came along in a variety of ways, some credible, more doubtful. I saw a number of Annie's classmates, many of whom considered her their "best friend." I wondered if Annie had the ability to allow others to think they were her best friends while not really letting them in. I wondered how I had failed to connect with her when so many peers seemed to have connected with her exceptionally well. Their level of grieving varied. Predictably, much of their grief was about themselves, their own doubts and fears. I began to wonder if my own unsettled feelings were about my own doubts and fears.

Her sister had information and insight. Annie had been using drugs the summer before. I learned that she had had sex with an older boy that summer. I found out that her parents had taken her to a couple of psychiatric hospitals for admittance last summer and were denied because the doctors thought that Annie's suicide threats were "attention seeking" rather than sincere. Perhaps Annie's dramatic presentation had contributed to her death by masking her symptoms, I thought.

I already knew that Annie had a history of running away. Her father had been struggling with a drinking problem and her mother had become more and more depressed and emotionally unavailable. The oldest sister, who still lived at home, was intact emotionally in spite of her own difficulties, and yet Annie had killed herself. What was the difference?

PSYCHOLOGICAL ANATOMY OF A GRIEVING THERAPIST

I began to realize that I was becoming obsessed with Annie's suicide. I had been processing frequently with colleagues and administrators as well as my multidisciplinary consultation team where I had presented the story of Annie. My clinical supervisor and clinic director provided a further clue. They very kindly confronted me about the fact that I, who work four-fifths time, had been putting in well over full-time hours. It was amazing to me that I didn't realize that I had been doing that for more than a month! I also had been unable to say "no" to seeing anyone, whereas previously I had good boundaries in terms of not taking too heavy of a client load. I even considered resigning from the state advisory subcommittee on children's mental health, which I very much enjoy. I felt that I was not really functioning very efficiently. It became obvious that, irrationally, I was punishing myself for failing to prevent Annie's suicide. Doing "penance" was better than feeling helpless and powerless. I realized that, more than anything, I wanted another chance with Annie.

Annie reminded me of my own children, whom I felt I could not bear to lose, even more so to suicide. (No one can bear to lose a child to suicide.) Annie's death reminded me of when my husband died suddenly of a heart attack when he was 43 and I was 34. Annie's death reminded me of when I was hospitalized for depression after an overdose when I was in my early twenties. I remembered feeling that I was in a narrow tunnel with only one option when I had overdosed. I have a faint memory of how very bad that felt, how bad it must have felt for Annie. Finally I had connected with her. Annie's death reminded me that there is so much that I cannot control.

WAYS I TRIED TO COPE AND THOSE WHO HELPED

I wrote poetry for Annie. In one poem I was very directive, talking to her standing on that chair with the noose around her neck. "You come down," I say and I fumble with giving her hope. Again and again I repeat, "You come down," but she ignores me. My directives strike me as very poor therapeutic style and largely maternal in tone. But Annie has no hope. In the poem she is done listening to me talk and she pushes away the chair and her life is over.

Another poem is called:

Portrait of a Family

Annie lies in her coffin, turtleneck sweater hiding the noose burns,
Mother worriedly brushes hair off Annie's forehead, pretending it matters,
Father paces, needing a drink,
Oldest sister socializes, trying to hold up the face of normalcy.
Shy sister hides in the back office of the church, her own terror closer,
The nine-year-old girl puts her favorite purple stuffed bear next to Annie,
watching for her to move,
Scared baby girl hovers near Mama, holding onto her skirt.
This is the family portrait; Annie is already 'hung.'

Finally my reaction began to feel more real. I realized that I had been in denial most of the time about the potential of a client I see, or have seen, completing suicide. I have always said that it is a risk therapists take and no one can prevent it from happening if a client is secret, hopeless and determined. But I never really believed it would happen to me. I pretended I had some mystical veil that protected me, or I imagined I was a magical healer who protected my clients, or some other self-protective nonsense. Never again will I be able to so completely deny the possibility.

E-mails to a good friend who is also a therapist were the most helpful to my healing. She had a way of reflecting back what she heard from me so that my understanding deepened. I had written that I felt like I was in outer space and that the rules of nature were not reliable. She responded,

"Oh, Gail, existential terror: the worst. It does seem like [Annie's] suicide ripped open your protective denial, that kind we all live with, the stance that makes it possible to live at all, the one that tells us that death is far away from us as individuals and that we have enough control to protect ourselves from this terrible thing. Children aren't supposed to die, especially by their own hand, and therefore it doesn't happen, not really, not to children we know, not to a child whom you held briefly in your grasp–that denial. The one that says that if we do our jobs responsibly and well and take care of our health and don't take unnecessary risks, well then, nothing awful will happen to us/those we care for professionally. The one that makes it possible to get up in the morning and breathe. (Hill, 2001)

Finally I was able to weep and I did so many times. When I realized that I would usually weep when my partner was available to comfort me, I took that as a sign I was healing. At least I had enough control in my life to time my grieving to coincide with receiving optimal comfort. I was coming toward some sort of acceptance.

I did not then know of the Website that addresses therapists' responses to the suicide of a client or patient by the American Association of Suicidology. That also would have helped and it has now. It is sponsored by the Clinician Survivor Task Force and can be found at <www.iusb.edu/~jmcintos/therapists_ mainpg.htm>.

HOW IS THIS ABOUT BEING FEMALE
FOR HER AND FOR ME?

It is easier to identify how Annie's death is related to her being female than it is to identify how my reactions to her death are about being female. Annie was not a survivor, but a victim of a society that doesn't value females who fail to follow gender-specific social rules. She got into fights in school, skipped school, used drugs and alcohol, and had sex at a young age. Her family held a history of intergenerational male-to-female abuse. She paid a high price for her behavioral "transgressions" and got called cruel sexist names like "whore" and "slut" when an older male used her sexually. Annie didn't believe that life was good because her life was not good in her estimation.

Annie grew to feel hopeless about therapy according to her sister. I learned that she had seen a couple of other therapists after me, never for long. Her sister said that Annie felt that no one understood her at a time in her life when she desperately needed affirmation. Another huge blow for her was the conflict between her parents and subsequent emotional loss of them, her father to alcohol and her mother to depression. This undercut any sense of security she had in her family. It also further undermined her trust in female/male relationships.

Unlike Annie, I came from an emotionally strong family, stable and well-educated. I am grateful that I have been encouraged to acknowledge and process my feelings with reasonable assurance that I can learn from my emotional pain and reach a place of resolution. I am grateful that I have a partner who values processing feelings. She can tolerate the discomfort of that process in her presence, and she knows how to comfort and nurture me. I am grateful that I have a good woman friend, who is also a therapist, who could be with me while I explored the agony of this experience. She skillfully walked the line between hearing me empathically and pushing me gently to the next questions in a warm and supportive way. I am grateful for my female supervisors who debriefed me more than once when I needed that. They understood that I needed to go to the wake and funeral. I learned later in my reading that reaching out to the family is advisable. "One of the greatest mistakes a therapist can make is to avoid the family, should the family seek the therapist out" (Ruben, 1990). My supervisors confronted me kindly when they saw that I had lost my boundaries. All of my colleagues, female and male, were willing to talk with me when I needed.

Probably the closest way I identified with Annie as another female is when I painfully remembered my overdose and hospitalization the day after I was raped because I was in the "wrong" place and didn't have a way to get home. For me that certainly was about being female and not feeling good enough about myself so that I took risks which made me vulnerable. It had been hard for me to forgive myself for my poor judgment in accepting a ride from a stranger. Yet I knew I did not want to be raped. That incident led to a year of intense therapy and ultimately a vocational choice. I chose to learn how to help others who need to be affirmed in their strengths and empowered to stop taking responsibility for abuse of power in a system which often rewards the aggressive and blames the innocent.

WHAT SELECTED LITERATURE SAYS
ABOUT THERAPIST AS SURVIVOR OF SUICIDE

Purposely I did not read the articles I had collected related to suicide of a client until I wrote my own story of Annie's suicide and how it had affected me. When I did read them, it was reassuring to find out how very typical my process was. Maltsberger (1992) suggests therapists "bereaved by suicide may respond with melancholia-like symptoms. Others develop atonement reactions marked by reaction formation and undoing. Others . . . exhibit avoidance reactions colored with denial, projection and distortion." Jones (1987) asserts that "the suicide of a patient in therapy is the most difficult bereavement crisis that a therapist will have to encounter and endure." Nor is such an experience rare in the world of therapists. A 1988 study by Chemtob, Hamada, Bauer, Torigoe, and Kinney found that of the 365 clinician respondents, 81 (22%) "reported having had a patient who committed suicide."

After reading about the experiences of other clinicians I learned how fortunate I was to not have to deal with the legal issues many face after the suicide of a client: issues of legal liability, questions of malpractice. "The grief and mourning of the therapist are important in that they obscure the matter of the therapist's role in the suicide" (Carter, 1971). Surely any fear of possible legal proceedings would have prevented the kind of open grieving process that I got to have, limited only by my insight and ability to process and still function.

I was further reinforced by a submission on the Suicidality Association's Website from an anonymous therapist: "There is no way for a good therapist to avoid the feelings of failure sooner or later." A November 2001 article in the American Psychological Association's *Monitor* on surviving a patient's suicide states ". . . therapists commonly cited sadness, depression, hopelessness, guilt and anger as reactions to a patient's suicide" in an unpublished study of 91 therapists conducted for the American Association of Suicidology (DeAngelis, 2001).

Feeling bad is much easier when I know that I am supposed to feel bad; I have permission to feel bad. Literature clearly supports that when therapists grieve personally for a client, we are like all other human beings and have very typical kinds of responses. We also tend to revisit old griefs when this loss touches our existential terror and the protective denial falls away temporarily. Maltsberger (1992) explains: "The sudden loss of a patient sometimes reactivates in the therapist an old depressive complex never before adequately resolved." "The adaptational challenge to any bereaved person is gradually to give up the defenses that are automatically called into play in the immediate experience of loss. In the acute situation, they are needed to ameliorate the flood of feelings that threaten to overwhelm," he writes.

Therapist stories and studies repeatedly point out that we have to do our personal grieving first before we can accurately assess our responsibility as therapists and all that entails. "Therefore, in the early phase of learning about the death of a patient, it is critically important for the therapist to gather all of the pertinent information about the suicide before reaching conclusions or making statements to others about the patient or his or her own role or responsibility relating to the patient's death" (Ruben, 1990). Talking with peers and supervisors who have had the experience and/or are willing to truly walk through the experience with therapists can lead us to have the courage to face our sense of failure, although that is not necessarily actual failure.

I was glad to hear that reaching out to the suicide victim's family is recommended and that attendance at the funeral is considered helpful (DeAngelis, 2001). I fumbled through the experience, got good help and now consider myself much closer to resolution. Beatrix Foster, a psychiatrist, wrote in 1987 that after the suicide of two patients, "I went to sleep, a sleep that lasted several months . . . And heal I did, though things are never quite the same." She refers to the "eternal problem of the patient's freedom [to complete suicide] and the therapist's power [limited by the patient's freedom to complete suicide]." She talks about the struggle of watching a patient grapple with suicidal wishes. "It demands much more of me, now that I know how it feels, to sit and witness the struggle between the choice of life and death. I know of no greater triumph than the choice for life made with just a glimmer of hope, apparently little to look forward to, when the choice to live is strictly a choice of risk and pain."

When the snow fell this fall, I thought of Annie's grave in the cemetery covered with snow, and I felt so very sad again. I think of her family and I quake for their loss. I have lost my innocence as a therapist. Annie lost her innocence as a girl a long time ago, and it killed her.

RESOLUTION AND TRANSFORMATION TO HOPE

Resolution and transformation are where I hope to land. I'm not quite there yet; that's why I'm writing this article. I'm worried about a feeling of distance I have more often now with clients. It is as if I don't dare care as much. For Annie's sake, I would like to care more than ever. That would be the best memorial I could construct. But I have to work out a balance between caring and my own lack of power to control the outcome; wise detachment from the outcome instead of anticipatory self-protection. Therapists craft the stuff of hope, and suicide sucks the life out of hope. I want to get back to hoping with abandon, but I'm not there yet. I'm still scared. Annie's hopelessness is eloquent, and it echoes in my ears, rings in my heart. Now that I finally connected with her, I don't want to disconnect, but I do want to completely detach from her choice of suicide. I want to fully engage, knowing I can't perfectly protect future Annies I might see.

The completed suicide of Annie took me through an initial denial and distancing and a gradual ownership that my reactions were in part about my own history of depression and losses, some gender-related. I was able to identify with Annie as a female who felt unvalidated at a critical time in her life and was exploited sexually. I recognize that I had many privileges she did not.

I grieve that she did not get meaningful help while I did. I lament the tragedy that she was loved and that was not enough for her to stay alive. The fact that I could not have prevented her suicide triggers my existential terror. I grieved the loss of Annie in the same manner all human beings grieve. I am working to not be fearful in therapy about losing clients to suicide because I want to be able to connect directly with them and offer them hope in a meaningful way.

In play therapy I often combine the wave of a magic wand with this phrase: "Love is stronger than hate, and good is more powerful than evil," words I believe on good days. To myself I add, "Hope is more potent than suicide."

REFERENCES

Carter, R.E. (1971). Some effects of client suicide on the therapist. *Psychotherapy: Theory, Research, and Practice, 8,* 287-289.

Chemtob, C.M., Hamada, R.S., Bauer, G., Torigoe, R.Y., & Kinney, B. (1988). Patients' suicides: Frequency and impact on psychiatrists. *American Journal of Psychiatry, 145,* 224-228.

DeAngelis, T. (2001, November). Surviving a patient's suicide. *APA Monitor,* 70-72, 75.

Foster, B. (1987). Suicide and the impact on the therapist. In J.L. Sacksteder, D.P. Schwartz & Y. Akabane (Eds.), *Attachment and the therapeutic process: Essays in honor of Otto Allen Will, Jr., M.D.,* 197-204. Madison, CT: International Universities Press.

Hill, M. (2001, June 6). Unpublished e-mail, personal communication.

Jones, F.A. Jr. (1987). Therapists as survivors of client suicide. In E.J. Dunne, J.L. McIntosh & K.L. Dunne-Maxim (Eds.), *Suicide and its aftermath: Understanding and counseling the survivors,* 126-141. New York: W.W. Norton.

Maltsberger, J.T. (1992). The implications of patient suicide for the surviving psychotherapist. In D. Jacobs (Ed.), *Suicide and clinical practice,* 169-182. Washington, DC: American Psychiatric Press, Clinical Practice No. 21.

Meade, J.F. (2001). American Association of Suicidology Clinician Survivor Task Force. <www.iusb.edu/~jmcintos/therapists_mainpg.htm>.

Ruben, H.L. (1990). Surviving a suicide in your practice. In S.J. Blumenthal & D.J. Kupfer (Eds.), *Suicide over the life cycle: Risk factors, assessment, and treatment of suicidal patients,* 619-636. Washington, DC: American Psychiatric Press.

Don't Forget About Me:
The Experiences of Therapists-in-Training
After a Client Has Attempted
or Died by Suicide

Jason S. Spiegelman
James L. Werth, Jr.

SUMMARY. The first half of this paper reviews the personal and professional experiences of the authors after having a client die by suicide

Jason S. Spiegelman received his BS in Psychology from the University of Pittsburgh in 1995, his MA in Clinical Psychology from Pepperdine University in 1997, and is currently a doctoral candidate in Counseling Psychology at the University of Akron. He has served on the boards of directors for the American Association of Suicidology (AAS) and the American Psychological Association, Division 12, Section VII (Clinical Emergencies and Crises). He is also a member of the AAS Clinician Survivor Task Force. He is currently employed as Adjunct Professor in the Department of Psychology at Towson University. A version of his personal story can be found on the Task Force's Website, which can be accessed through <www.suicidology.org> or directly at <www.iusb.edu/~jmcintos/therapists_mainpg.htm>.

James L. Werth, Jr., received a PhD in Counseling Psychology from Auburn University in 1995 and a Masters of Legal Studies from the University of Nebraska-Lincoln in 1999. He has been employed as Assistant Professor in the Department of Psychology at The University of Akron since August 2000. He also is a member of the AAS Clinician Survivor Task Force.

Address correspondence to: James L. Werth, Jr., Department of Psychology, The University of Akron, Akron, OH 44325-4301 (E-mail: jwerth@uakron.edu).

[Haworth co-indexing entry note]: "Don't Forget About Me: The Experiences of Therapists-in-Training After a Client Has Attempted or Died by Suicide." Spiegelman, Jason S., and James L. Werth, Jr. Co-published simultaneously in *Women & Therapy* (The Haworth Press, Inc.) Vol. 28, No. 1, 2005, pp. 35-57; and: *Therapeutic and Legal Issues for Therapists Who Have Survived a Client Suicide: Breaking the Silence* (ed: Kayla Miriyam Weiner) The Haworth Press, Inc., 2005, pp. 35-57. Single or multiple copies of this article are available for a fee from The Haworth Document Delivery Service [1-800-HAWORTH, 9:00 a.m. - 5:00 p.m. (EST). E-mail address: docdelivery@haworthpress.com].

Digital Object Identifier: 10.1300/J015v28n01_04

(the first author) or make a serious attempt (the second author). The second half reviews research on training and graduate students' experience with suicide and attempted suicide and then reviews supervisors' interventions. The paper ends with sets of suggestions for trainees, supervisors, and clinical programs. *[Article copies available for a fee from The Haworth Document Delivery Service: 1-800-HAWORTH. E-mail address: <docdelivery@haworthpress.com> Website: <http://www.HaworthPress.com> © 2005 by The Haworth Press, Inc. All rights reserved.]*

KEYWORDS. Graduate students, training, suicide, attempted suicide, supervision

INTRODUCTION

The title of this paper is a request on two levels: (a) that graduate students not be forgotten in the discussion about the aftereffects of a client's suicidality, and (b) that recognition be given to the toll that an attempted suicide can take on the clinician. Although the effects of completed suicide on professional therapists are not to be minimized, we want to ensure that trainees and professional therapists whose clients attempt but do not complete suicide are not inadvertently omitted from consideration.

During the authors' practica experiences, the first author experienced the death of a client by suicide and the second author had a client make a serious attempt (see DeAngelis, 2001; Spiegelman, 2001). We will base the first half of this paper on those experiences, providing a review of the cases, our internal and external processing at the time, and the lasting effects the experiences have had on us both in our clinical work, our training and supervisory efforts, and our personal lives.

The second half of the paper will review research on training in suicidality in graduate training programs, graduate students' experience with suicide and attempted suicide, and the personal and professional consequences of these events on therapists-in-training. In addition, we will review supervisory interventions discussed in the literature and highlight legal and ethical considerations. We close with suggestions for trainees, supervisors, and clinical programs. These suggestions will be based on both our own experiences and the discussion in the literature.

CASE 1: DEATH BY SUICIDE

The purpose of this section is to familiarize the reader with the experience that the first author had with losing a client to suicide during his training years. The highly personal nature of this experience demands that such an account be given in the first person. In both this and the following accounts, the clients' identifying information has been masked to protect their confidentiality.

Background

I was near the end of my first practicum experience, and was within sight of the completion of my Master's degree. I had been seeing the same clients in therapy for several months, having worked at the same site for nearly 14 months, and I was confident that the termination sessions, which would begin in six weeks, would go smoothly. The impression I had when I left on a weekend trip was that my clients had, for the most part, improved, and those who had not had certainly not deteriorated. I had no inkling of the reality of the situation that would blindside me.

I had been seeing "Paul," a thirty-something client, for approximately four months. He had been a client of the clinic for many years and had seen several counselors and psychiatrists during his time there. He had availed himself of virtually every program offered via the clinic, but had experienced little appreciable improvement. His multiaxial diagnosis was a complex mix of psychosis- and anxiety-related symptoms, and his medical history included conditions that had left him with residual brain impairment. He was a tough client–he was my client.

The one thread of consistency that had plagued Paul over the course of his life was the feeling that he was "a burden to [his] family" and that he would be better off dead. No logical argument from clinician or relative could dissuade him from this position; in fact, no argument was needed. I believe that arguing illogical stances with logical reasoning is a futile effort, and it is a trap into which I often fell with Paul.

Despite my constant monitoring of Paul's suicidality–which revealed an ever-present ideation but an absence of any formalized plan, history of attempts, or palpable intent–Paul decided to take his own life. He bought flowers and went to visit the gravesite of his deceased mother. He went home when he knew his father would not be there, stepped into the backyard, and hung himself from the overhead deck that he and his father had built together. He left no note for his father but, in the weeks that followed, his father came to understand that the bouquet of flowers that Paul had left at his mother's headstone was a message more clear than any he could have put on paper. It was his final attempt to communicate that his anguish over both his mother's death and his own personal difficulties had become too much to bear. The flowers also represented Paul's final apology to his father, to whom he had so often begged for forgiveness for being a burden.

Personal Reaction

I found out that Paul had taken his life when I returned to the clinic after my weekend sojourn. I walked in to gather my messages and pull charts for the day's clients, and the receptionist informed me that a client of mine had suicided and that I was expected in the office of the clinical director (who was not my supervisor). The moments that followed are no longer clear to me, despite the fact that it has only been five years. The one reaction that does stand out, however, was my immediate thought that "this has to be a joke." Surely I would not have been told this news by the receptionist! "Where was my supervisor?" "Why wasn't I called at home?" And, of course, "Why do they want to see me? Do they think that it's my fault?"

The walk up to the second floor was the loneliest of my life, and the sound of my footfalls on the concrete steps reverberating through the brick-encased stairwell echo in my memory. I was gripped with an immediate need to use the bathroom, though I was more aware of the nausea that was building inside of me. A torrent of thoughts raced through my head as I considered the implications of the news that I had received. I felt a terrible sense of loss, for both the client's father and myself. I felt tremendous doubt in my own competence as a counselor and at the same time I felt angry with Paul for making this decision that so hurt everyone in his life. I felt terribly afraid for the consequences that I would have to face, and I also felt a horrible sense of guilt for the selfishness that I was displaying. "How can you think about your career," I asked myself. "Your client killed himself!" The emotions were numerous–far too many to be documented here–but the one that stands out in my mind is the pervasive feeling I had of being alone. I was very aware that for the next several minutes I was going to be standing on my own, a virtual child in the very adult world of psychology.

Supervisors' and Peers' Reactions

My loneliness was really nobody's fault. Both my immediate supervisor and my secondary supervisor (Paul's psychiatrist) were out of town on family emergencies. Neither had been informed of the suicide, and thus, neither was able to advocate for me, even from afar. The main reaction that I had to face was that of the clinic administrator(s). Both the director and the assistant director of the clinic were concerned about the potential repercussions of a client suicide, and their concerns were justifiably amplified by the fact that the deceased was a client of a trainee. Despite the weekly meetings that I had with both my supervisor and the client's psychiatrist, there was still a fear that the clinic would be implicated in the death. Given this fear, Brown's (1989) assertion that we must avoid engaging in either a "witchhunt or a whitewash" (p. 429) of trainees who have lost a client to suicide became particularly salient.

The questions that I answered in the hours that followed had an edge to them. I had an unmistakable sense that every aspect of the client's case was being scrutinized and there were poorly veiled threats that I would be held responsible for any mistakes that were found in my work. I was denied permission to review the case file, forbidden to contact Paul's father to convey condolences (a decision that was eventually reversed), and asked about every conceivable detail of the manner in which I had tracked, assessed, and consulted around the client's chronic suicidality.

The most difficult part of the experience was the urgency associated with the questions. When I asked the assistant director for time to talk to my supervisor before I spoke further with her, the response was, "We can't wait for him to get back into town. You have to answer these questions now." Faced with such haste I did the only thing I thought I could–I complied!

By the time my supervisor returned to town, the damage to my confidence as a therapist-in-training had been done. He informed me that he thought I was a talented and competent young clinician who had a bright future ahead of me, and reassured me that all of the proper steps had been taken with regard to Paul. Despite the very supportive nature of his comments, they provided only a small amount of ephemeral comfort.

The response from my academic department was far less pejorative, though equally unsupportive. I was passed from professor to professor as each was unwilling or unable to take the time I needed to allow me to process the events. When the suicide was brought up in my weekly practicum meeting, I was given just a few moments to talk about the event before we were urged to move on to the next student and the next case. There was no time given to my personal feelings of shame, anger, fear, or guilt. All was handled with a clinical efficiency that seemed quite out of place in a psychology program. I vividly recall the sense of frustration and disappointment that I felt leaving the class, as I had hoped that it would be a respite from my sense of being unsupported by professionals at the clinic.

One saving grace was the friendship and support of the other students in my program. Conversations during lunch breaks or over coffee, telephone calls, and the occasional card gave me the support that I craved. These responses let me know that I was not alone and that my peers shared my experience vicariously.

Effects on Professional Development

Although the suicide of one of my clients occurred in the last semester of my Master's training, I did not seriously address the feelings until well into my doctoral work. It was not until a supervisor noticed that I was avoiding certain types of clients–those who appeared to be even moderately depressed on intake–that I came face-to-face with my fear. It took that observation for me to realize that I was fleeing from clinical contact with any individuals who might have been a threat to engage in self-injurious behaviors.

Acknowledging the fear that was keeping me from these clients, I threw myself into the activities that would ultimately be the most useful in my own "recovery." I sought a personal counselor so that I could finally unload the burden of the feelings that I had never felt free to share. I wrote about my experiences in my practicum journal, though ultimately I decided that those entries were for my eyes only. I was fortuitously assigned to work as a graduate assistant for a professor who had an interest in clinical suicidology, and with his encouragement I began to write about my experiences and present on them at national conferences (e.g., Spiegelman, 2001; Spiegelman & Rogers, 2000). Through these presentations and publications I discovered that there are others who have struggled with the same issues, the same questions, and the same doubts. Ultimately the experience has become a driving force in my developing career, and though I would not wish such a devastating event on any young therapist, the reality that clients of graduate students will kill themselves means that we need to address rather than avoid the issue of client suicide during the training years.

CASE 2: ATTEMPTED SUICIDE

In this section the second author describes his experience with a female client's serious attempt at suicide while he was a trainee at a university counseling center. As with case 1, it will be written in the first person to highlight the personal nature of the episode and its effects.

Background

I was a fairly confident practicum student, even though I was in the early years of my graduate program, having been trained as a paraprofessional peer counselor and a suicide hotline volunteer as an undergraduate. I had had good experiences with clients, and I trusted myself and my supervisors. Therefore, I believed I could help the newest client assigned to me, "Audrey," with her self-esteem and eating-related concerns.

Over the course of six sessions we developed what I considered to be a good therapeutic alliance, and we seemed to be making progress. My site supervisor at the time had expertise in eating disorders, so I knew I was getting good supervision that was helping me help the client with her bulimia. We got to the point where she decided to not binge-and-purge between sessions. We had worked a little on coping mechanisms, and she had successfully implemented some in the face of triggers over the previous weeks. I remember feeling proud and excited as she left the session that day, looking forward to telling my supervisor and awaiting word the next week about whether she had met her goal.

However, the next week she did not show for her session nor did she call. This was unusual, as she had never even been late before. I followed standard protocol in such situations and talked about it with my site supervisor. She said we did not seem to have any reason to be concerned. The following week Audrey came in for her regular appointment–I had held the slot for her–and even in the waiting room she did not seem the same as she had two weeks earlier. As soon as the office door closed, she apologized for missing the previous week and not calling. She said she was in the hospital after attempting suicide following a breakup with her boyfriend.

Personal Reaction

I vividly recall that moment. I can remember what the room looked like, where the chairs were placed, what I was wearing, what she was wearing. I also remember the feeling, and I get shivers to this day. I was stunned silent in my sense of overwhelm, shock, and horror. I am sure I did not manage my non-verbal communication well, as she immediately said it was not my fault. Today I cannot recall the details of the session after that, even though I listened to the tape several times afterward, but I remember having many thoughts racing through my head and many questions, most that were probably irrational and all of which placed the responsibility on myself: "What did I miss?" "How could I have prevented this?" "What did I do wrong?" "What if she had died?" "What do I do now?" "I must be incompetent." "I almost killed her." "I better not see her or any other clients because I may hurt them." "What will my supervisors say?" "What will my peers think?" "Will I be kicked out of the program?" "Will the counseling center director cancel my practicum placement?" "Will I be sued?" . . .

I somehow made it through the session, probably relying on foundational counseling skills like reflections and minimal encouragers, and immediately sought out my site supervisor. She was in session, but the center director was available. I sat down and began babbling. I believe that without his support and that of my site supervisor, departmental supervisor, and classmates/other counseling center practicum trainees, I might have quit. It was devastating.

Supervisors' and Peers' Reactions

I do not remember exactly what the director did or said, but he calmed me. He had supervised me before, so he reassured me that I had done good work previously and that he was sure that my current supervisor would have let me know if what I was doing was problematic or counterproductive. He also said that we couldn't take responsibility for our clients' every decision. Finally, he told me that I should have the remainder of my clients that day cancelled and rescheduled for the following week but that I was in no danger of losing my placement.

Then my on-site supervisor and I met for over an hour with me summarizing what had happened, talking about how I felt, asking questions, and expressing self-doubts. She reminded me that she had closely supervised me with this client, had listened to tapes, and had reviewed my case conceptualization and interventions; however, she had not anticipated this happening. The fact that eating disorders were her area of specialization helped, but I still had doubts. She then said the same thing the director had said–we do not have control over our clients' lives and therefore cannot hold ourselves responsible for their decisions.

I went to my department that afternoon for my weekly group supervision with my departmental supervisor and my three peers (it just happened to be scheduled on the day I saw Audrey). I told my departmental supervisor beforehand what had happened, and he allowed me to use the entire two-hour session to talk and to get support from him and my peers. They all were very reassuring, as were the other students doing their practica at the counseling center, when they heard. I feel very fortunate to not have anyone even remotely hint that I was to blame for the suicide attempt.

Effects on Professional Development

Although everyone was doing her or his best to keep me from taking responsibility for Audrey's suicide attempt, as strange as it may sound, I think I wanted to find a way to make it my "fault." There was a part of me that thought if it was something I did or didn't do that caused the attempt, then I just needed to do something different so that it wouldn't happen again with another client–if it was under my control then I could keep any other client from attempting or completing suicide.

Another way of coping for me was to see if I was–as I believed–the only one who had had this happen. What I found was that it actually was not rare for a trainee to have someone die by suicide, let alone attempt it. This spurred me on, and I tried to find everything I could about the incidence and effects of client suicide on trainees and professionals. I wrote papers and gave presentations in graduate school. This continued in internship, where I remember one of my fellow interns saying, "This really affected you, even years later I can hear it in your voice as you talk about it with us." Even after graduation and when I started supervising trainees, first in a university counseling center and now in a departmental training clinic, I make it a point to talk to my supervisees about suicide, the possibility of having a client attempt or die by suicide, and make sure they know that I will support them if this happens. I also share my own experience.

I realize that the experience has shaped my view of my roles and responsibilities as a counselor and my client's roles and responsibilities. My outlook on life is probably related to going through this, as I have a strong need for control over my own life but also have a strong sense that I have little control over others. Many events have shaped who I am today as a person and as a professional; however, few other experiences are as seared into my brain as sitting with Audrey that day.

LITERATURE REVIEW ON TRAINEES
AND SUICIDE/ATTEMPTED SUICIDE

Training on Suicidality

Despite consistently reported findings that attempted or completed suicide by clients are very real phenomena that occur in all arenas of professional mental health, including psychiatry (Chemtob, Hamada, Bauer, Kinney, & Torigoe, 1988), psychology (Chemtob, Hamada, Bauer, Torigoe, & Kinney, 1988), social work and nursing (Brown, 1989), and further indications that the suicide or attempted suicide of a client is among the most potentially damaging to an individual's personal and professional sense of self (e.g., Brown, 1987, 1989; Chemtob, Hamada, Bauer, Kinney, & Torigoe, 1988; Chemtob, Hamada, Bauer, Torigoe, & Kinney, 1988; Deutsch, 1984; Goldstein & Buongiorno, 1984; Jobes & Maltsberger, 1995; Kleespies, 1993; Kleespies, Penk, & Forsyth, 1993; Kleespies, Smith, & Becker, 1990; Kozlowska, Nunn, & Cousens; 1997; Ruben, 1990; Shein, 1976; Valente, 1994), the issue of client suicidality and appropriate clinical and programmatic response is underrepresented in the literature. Given this assertion, it is also likely that the issue is also given inadequate attention in practice.

For at least 25 years authors have noted that both clinician-trainees and professionals are being left to their own resources when it comes to dealing with client suicidality (Shein, 1976). Although students are advised of their legal and ethical responsibilities in the case of potential imminent self-harm of their clients (they need to practice up to the "standard of care"–see, e.g., Bongar, 2002), the responses beyond the acute crisis situation are often neglected. Bongar and Harmatz (1989) and Brown (1989) both called for increased attention to the study of suicide during the graduate training years, and Brown further challenged the field to institute formal programmatic responses to trainees who have suffered a client suicide. Bongar and Harmatz reported that just over one-third of clinical psychology programs surveyed offered any formal didactic training in suicide issues, and further noted that "if training occurred, it was usually offered as part of another course" (p. 209).

Despite the findings, a recent investigation by Ellis and Dickey (1998) indicates that challenges to change these trends have gone unanswered. They found that the primary method for addressing suicidality in clients is via supervision. This suggests that there is still a trend of avoiding the issue until it presents in a clinical setting. Ellis and Dickey also report that where didactic training (e.g., workshops) are in place, they "were offered by only about half of psychology programs" (p. 493). It appears as if graduate psychology training programs are content with the status quo of suicide training despite narrative evidence that such failures to establish this important clinical training area are potentially detrimental to developing professional therapists (Brown, 1987; Brown, 1989, Kleespies, 1993; Kleespies, Penk, & Forsyth, 1993; Kleespies,

Smith, & Becker, 1990; Kolodny et al., 1979; Spiegelman, 2001; Spiegelman & Rogers, 2000).

The training that appears to be most readily available to students comes during the practical training phases, when students are engaged in practica or even predoctoral internships or postdoctoral fellowships (Ellis & Dickey, 1998). The Association of Psychology Postdoctoral and Internship Centers (APPIC) publishes information about those training sites where a student may expect some informal or formal rotation in "crisis intervention." The American Psychological Association, Division 12, Section VII (Clinical Emergencies and Crises) is currently engaged in a research effort to identify other training sites where formalized practical education in crisis intervention is available.

Although these are steps in the right direction, they highlight the larger problem that most students are ill-prepared for such experiences coming out of their academic training years. We believe it is irresponsible of academic programs to send students to external practica or internships with only the minimal skills needed to deal with suicidal clients, a situation akin to teaching someone to swim only after she or he has been thrown into deep water. It is not sufficient to teach a therapist-in-training to perform a skeletal suicide assessment without preparing her or him for the possibility that the client will attempt, or worse yet die by, suicide. Students can be left with the feeling that suicide is something that happens to other clinicians, and certainly not to trainees, and thus hide behind the thin veil of denial that it is a potential hurdle that they will have to overcome in their own career. Suicide as a clinical possibility is something that must be demystified and brought into the collective conscious of training programs.

Incidence of Experience with Suicide/Attempted Suicide

The current available research has documented the extent, and potentially severe effects, of client suicidal actions on therapists-in-training. In their survey of psychology interns and trainees, Kleespies, Penk, and Forsyth (1993) found that approximately 1 in 9 of their respondents had a client die by suicide and almost 1 in 4 had a client attempt suicide during their years as psychologists-in-training. In addition, Kleespies (1993, p. 477) stated that "psychologists in training have an acute reaction to patient suicide that is at least as strong, if not stronger, than their professional counterparts." When suicidal gestures–attempts and completions–are viewed together, Kleespies (1993) reports that an estimated 40% of trainees will deal with suicidal clients in some form over the course of their clinical training years.

Kleespies and colleagues (1993) examined various factors that may have been associated with a trainee's likelihood of experiencing client suicidality and found no significant differences between trainees based on age, sex, or years of training. Although one might intuitively think that more advanced trainees would be more likely to encounter client suicidality, as trainees with less experience might be prevented from taking more complex cases, this was not the case. Surprisingly, this absence of training effect does not persist in the research with professional therapists. Chemtob and his colleagues (Chemtob, Hamada, Bauer, Kinney, & Torigoe, 1988; Chemtob, Hamada, Bauer, Torigoe, & Kinney, 1988) found a significant inverse relationship between years of training and likelihood of experiencing a client suicide for both professional psychologists and psychiatrists. They did not find, however, that years of *practice* had the same insulating effect for professional psychologists. In other words, it appears that experience as a clinician is less important than the quality and quantity of training that a psychologist receives regarding appropriate and effective ways of responding to a potentially suicidal client. These data regarding professional mental health providers further support claims that training in client suicidality at the graduate, and even postgraduate level, is crucial.

Kleespies and his coauthors (1993) documented that there are no significant gender differences in how trainees responded to suicide attempts or completions but that there was a significant increase in scores on the Impact of Events Scale (IES) for both those who had a client attempt or complete suicide. Furthermore, there was a significant difference between these two groups on one of the three IES subscales—those trainees who had a client complete suicide were more significantly impacted on the Avoidance subscale of the IES, a measure that describes an individual's attempts to minimize or steer clear of thoughts related to the event in question. For the clinician-in-training, this might translate into actions that decrease the student's willingness to work with suicidal clients in the future, to process the event in supervision, or to seek out those avenues of remediation that might cause the trainee to face the events on a repeated basis. These avoidant behaviors, if not curtailed, can lead to serious restrictions for a developing career. Further, the longer the delay in addressing the consequences, the more difficult it may eventually be to reverse the negative effects of such a clinical event.

Personal and Professional Consequences

Research investigating the effects of client suicidal behaviors on clinicians-in-training is relatively scarce, as more attention has been paid to the effects on mental health professionals. Many have argued (Brown, 1989; Kleespies, 1993; Kleespies et al., 1993; Lynch, 1987; Spiegelman, Ellis, Briggs, & Rogers, 2000) that the effects noted with established professional providers are all potential consequences for the trainee. In addition, the trainee must grapple with additional concerns, including worries over negative evaluative outcomes, suspension or termination from clinical sites or training programs, and interruption of degree attainment. These worries, which carry among them the common theme of blame, are alluded to by Jobes and Maltsberger (1995) who note that "the suicide death of a patient in active treatment is commonly taken as prima facie evidence that the therapist, somehow or another, has mismanaged the case" (pp. 200-201), and that even though suicide occurs despite the best efforts to prevent it, "too often, the scapegoat selected is the clinician who was trying to treat the illness and prevent the suicide" (p. 201).

In terms of long-term effects, Kleespies (1993, p. 480) quoted two student-respondents who said, respectively, "I think it certainly had a significant impact . . . For a year I didn't want to be a therapist. I didn't do work on the inpatient unit for a year, partly by choice . . ." and "It had a very profound impact. I debated getting out of this work. It was hard to talk about it. I felt a tremendous amount of responsibility. I felt a real sense of loss. . . . I'm still scared by it. What would it mean if it happened again?" Such findings have important implications when examined in light of the numbers of trainees who have clients attempt or die by suicide.

Lynch (1987) points out that the trainee has a personal investment in being viewed by her or his supervisors, peers, and colleagues as being capable and skilled to provide the services of a therapist: "There is a great value attached to wanting to be seen by one's patients and one's supervisors as highly compassionate, caring, non-rejecting, [and] non-punitive" (p. 100). This statement speaks to the very heart of the issue of client suicidal behavior–the potential damage to the trainee's perception of her or his own competence to perform continued psychotherapy, particularly given the likelihood that she or he will deal with client suicidality in the future. As both authors have indicated above, even the possibility of a client suicide caused an anxious examination of our career choice, competence, and willingness to engage in future counseling with potentially suicidal clients.

Little attention has been paid to the personal effects of client suicidality on the clinician-in-training. What little research is available has again focused on the professional therapist. Chemtob and his colleagues (Chemtob, Hamada, Bauer, Kinney, & Torigoe, 1988; Chemtob, Hamada, Bauer, Torigoe, & Kinney, 1988) have indicated that professional therapists experience personal consequences severe enough to approximate the response to the death of a parent. Although it cannot be stated that a trainee in the same situation will have an identical level of response, it may be inferred from the literature that equates the responses of trainees to the responses of professionals that such a personal impact on the trainee is possible, and even likely (Kleespies et al., 1990, 1993).

Supervisory Interventions Discussed in the Literature

A variety of authors have discussed the effects of suicide or attempted suicide on therapists and trainees, and many of these articles have included discussions of what supervisors, colleagues, and employers can do to assist the clinician/student (e.g., Jones, 1987; Kleespies, 1993; Valente, 1994). This section will briefly highlight those interventions that are most commonly mentioned and have been demonstrated in the research to be most helpful. Because of the relatively small literature base on trainees, we will also draw from material on professional therapists. We also note that some authors highlighted a developmental process involving a "working through" of the attempt/death, so considering how different interventions may be more useful at different phases may be important (e.g., Brown, 1989; Carter, 1971; Goldstein & Buongiorno, 1984; Kleespies, 1993; Kolodny, Binder, Bronstein, & Friend, 1979; Marshall, 1980; Menninger, 1991; Tanney, 1995). Finally, we need to mention that we are focusing on a suicide attempt or death that occurs with a client who is being seen in individual counseling in an outpatient setting; if the client was part of a group or in an inpatient facility then there are additional considerations regarding the trainee's responsibilities to the other group members and inpatient clients that are too complex to discuss here.

Several authors (e.g., Carter, 1971; Marshall, 1980; Ruben, 1990) focused on the need for the therapist to gather information about the suicide (we would say the same is true for attempts), preferably from a neutral source (e.g., a coroner). However, there are some cautions about discussing the case with others (see next section).

Many articles emphasized the need for the clinician/trainee to get formal support from supervisors or senior colleagues as well as informal assistance from the therapist's/student's significant others (e.g., Brown, 1989; Carter, 1971; Kleespies et al., 1990, 1993). Other sources emphasized that during this meeting with a supervisor or colleague, responsibility for the attempt or death should not be assigned by the supervisor but instead the person should receive reassurance (e.g., Carter, 1971; Ellis & Dickey, 1998; Feldman, 1987; Kaye & Soreff, 1991; Kleespies, 1993; Kleespies, Niles, Mori, & Deleppo, 1998). Meanwhile, Bongar (2002), coming from a risk management perspective, urged those involved in a situation where someone has died to immediately consult with an attorney–a procedure which could obviously increase the stress and sensitivity of all involved. During the immediate phase it may also be helpful for the trainee to know that she or he is not the only one who has had a client attempt or die by suicide. In addition, supervisors need to continue to work with students as they deal with the death (or attempt) and help the trainee determine how, if at all, the experience is affecting work with other clients (Brown; Feldman; Kleespies).

Perhaps the most frequent ongoing intervention suggested is providing for individual discussion and, if possible, group support (e.g., Alexander, Klein, Gray, Dewar, & Eagles, 2000; Brown, 1989; Feldman, 1987; Goldstein & Buongiorno, 1984; Holden, 1978; Jones, 1987; Kaye & Soreff, 1991; Kleespies, 1993; Kleespies et al., 1990, 1993, 1998; Kolodny et al., 1979; Marshall, 1980; Menninger, 1991; Ruben, 1990; Valente, 1994). Tanney (1995) suggested that not only should there be an informal forum, a consultant should be available for a year (see also, Brown; Marshall). Some trainees/therapists may want to pursue their own counseling (Brown; Ellis & Dickey, 1998; Kleespies et al., 1993; Ruben).

Kolodny and colleagues (1979) described their experiences as trainees who all had a client die by suicide during the same spring and how they coped individually and as a group–using each other for support (see also Feldman, 1987). Jones (1987) provided the most complete discussion of how a support group can be useful for therapists as well as collateral personnel when a client dies by suicide. More formal meetings such as case conferences or "psychological autopsies" can also be helpful if the focus is on learning as opposed to assigning blame (Alexander et al., 2000; Brown, 1989; Ellis & Dickey, 1998; Kaye & Soreff, 1991; Kleespies, 1993; Kleespies et al., 1990, 1993, 1998; Marshall, 1980; Tanney, 1995; Valente, 1994).

Other types of interventions include attending the funeral, wake, or other ritual if the client died; and meeting with the significant others of the person who attempted/died, perhaps with another therapist present (Alexander et al., 2000; Bongar, 2002; Brown, 1989; Holden, 1978; Jones, 1987; Kaye & Soreff, 1991; Kleespies, 1993; Kleespies et al., 1990, 1993, 1998; Menninger, 1991; Tanney, 1995; Valente, 1994)–although this meeting must be carefully managed (see below).

Many authors also emphasized that the therapist/trainee will likely experience a sense of grief and/or guilt (e.g., Carter, 1971; Feldman, 1987; Goldstein & Buongiorno, 1984; Kleespies, 1993; Kolodny et al., 1979; Marshall, 1980; Ruben, 1990; Valente, 1994). Grief can be considered natural, but guilt can complicate resolution of grief–although the research indicates that it is a natural reaction, given the relationship of the client and trainee/therapist. Therefore, perhaps the best intervention is providing graduate students training about suicide, the possibility that they will have a client attempt or complete suicide, and what typical reactions are, before they experience such an event (e.g., Kleespies, 1993; Kleespies et al., 1990, 1993, 1998; Menninger, 1991; see also Brown, 1989; Jones, 1987; Marshall). Such education may prevent excessive guilt and enable trainees to seek and receive support from peers and supervisors.

Finally, several sources emphasized the need for treatment settings to have established guidelines for what to do in the event of a suicide attempt or death (e.g., Ellis & Dickey, 1998; Kaye & Soreff, 1991; Kleespies et al., 1998; Marshall, 1980; Menninger, 1991; for guidelines about handling suicidal clients before an attempt or death, see Jobes & Berman, 1993). Suggestions for such guidelines are provided in the final section of this paper.

Legal and Ethical Issues

Although some actions to assist the trainee who has had a client attempt or complete suicide may seem to be common sense, there may be negative ramifications if action is taken too quickly, without considering the ethical and legal implications. Unfortunately, there is not as much material available on this subject as there is on potential interventions (although there is some information on risk management when working with clients who are suicidal, see, e.g., Bongar, 2002; Bongar, Berman et al., 1998).

Fear of being sued is a common reaction to a death (Kleespies et al., 1998; Litman, 1965) and may be similarly so after an attempt. This is legitimate concern, given the reports which indicate that "malpractice related to suicide is the sixth most frequent claim brought against psychologists [and it is] the second most costly" (Jobes & Berman, 1993, p. 92; Bongar, Maris, Berman, & Litman, 1998). Recent events at the Massachusetts Institute of Technology (MIT) counseling center, in which the parents of a client who committed suicide are suing the institution, highlight this issue.

In training situations, students are not the ones truly at risk, as their supervisors bear the ultimate responsibility (Bongar, Maris et al., 1998; Ellis & Dickey, 1998). Thus, it behooves the trainee and supervisor both to be careful about what is said and done following a death or attempt, so as not to unintentionally implicate oneself or another as a "cause" of the client's action. This is especially important given the suggestions in the literature that trainees/therapists seek information and perhaps meet with loved ones of the person who attempted or died (e.g., Carter, 1971; Kaye & Soreff, 1991; Ruben, 1990). Some have asserted that meeting with family members may reduce the threat of a malpractice suit (e.g., Bongar, 2002). However, the therapist/trainee must walk a fine line in such meetings, as the confidentiality of the client who attempted or completed suicide must be protected (Bongar; Werth, Burke, & Bardash, 2002).

Several authors have noted that malpractice claims against treating mental health personnel after a suicide are often born out of anger and guilt felt by loved ones and displaced onto the treaters, who were supposed to have prevented the attempt or death from happening (e.g., Bongar, 2002; Ruben, 1990). This may be even more likely in situations where the client was seeing a trainee–loved ones may assume there was substandard care and "if only" the person had been seeing a "professional" the attempt or death would not have happened (Bongar, Maris et al., 1998; Ruben). This possibility, therefore, makes it clear that both supervisors and students need to have adequate training in suicide assessment and intervention; that the supervisor attempt to ensure that the student is assigned appropriate clients given her or his level of skill and experience; that there is a signed informed consent from the client regarding receiving care from a trainee; and that the student and supervisor both consult regularly and document thoroughly (Bongar; Bongar, Maris et al.; Ellis & Dickey, 1998; Packman & Harris, 1998). In addition, supervisors must make sure that trainees attempt to get prior treatment records if the client reports having received mental health services in the past (Packman & Harris).

One final consideration is the confidentiality of the supervisory sessions and notes in the event that there is an ethical or legal claim brought against the trainee, and therefore the supervisor (Ellis & Dickey, 1998). Bongar (2002; see also Ruben, 1990) warned that professionals should be careful about what they say and to whom, as anyone could be subpoenaed to testify, and should only discuss possible errors in their personal psychotherapy or with an attorney (both of these situations allow the therapist to invoke privilege). In addition, there may be situations where the institution has created safeguards related to access and use of confidential information, such as what may be discussed in a peer review or quality assurance meeting (Bongar; Ellis & Dickey). The question then arises as to whether supervision, as well as psychological autopsies or other individual/group meetings related where the incident is discussed, could also be considered to allow for privilege. Ellis and Dickey concluded that "there seems to be no current legal precedent for a supervisor's being required to divulge the content of a post-suicide debriefing in malpractice proceedings" (p. 496). These authors also emphasized that although there may be concern about discussing the suicide or attempt, a program might be at equal or greater legal risk by *not* pursuing all reasonable means to understand the course of events leading to a patient's suicide and endeavoring to correct any deficiencies that may be identified, either in the program or within the trainee. The question therefore becomes whether a clinical training site has an ethical responsibility to utilize a negative therapeutic outcome–attempted or completed suicide–in a manner that will be educative to the therapist-trainees, and if so, whether this obligation supersedes the clinic's/program's justifiable concern over exposing itself to potential lawsuits in the wake of such an incident.

We believe that although confidentiality is a consideration, both with loved ones of the person who attempted or died by suicide, as well as with people who could be subpoenaed if a legal (or ethical) case is brought, fear of reprisal should not prevent a supervisor or training program from attending to the emotional and training needs of a student.

SUGGESTIONS FOR TRAINING AND FOR SUPERVISORS

Based on the material reviewed above and our own experiences, we provide several suggestions for what trainees, supervisors, and training sites/programs can do following a suicide attempt or death by a student's client. The recommendations provided below should be viewed with three considerations in mind. First, it should be noted that all of the suggestions–to trainees, supervisors, and programs–are made with the assumption that client confidentiality will always be given requisite consideration. For example, if inquiries or contacts are to be made, they must be done so with the client's privacy respected to the greatest extent possible. Second, the proposals which encourage open communication between a trainee and her or his supervisor(s) should all be considered while bearing in mind Bongar's (2002) cautions regarding the privilege, or lack thereof, of such conversations. Finally, where possible, these lists are organized with a temporal sequence kept in mind, so that trainees, supervisors, and program administrators can utilize them before an attempted or completed suicide occurs, immediately after, and between three and six months following such an event.

Trainees

1. As soon as possible, meet with your immediate supervisor or if this person is unavailable, another supervisor at the site/in your department; try not talk to others about what happened until you can confer with a supervisor.
2. Bring the client file and any audio-/videotapes to a meeting with your supervisor.
3. If your supervisor allows, tell her or him your emotional reaction to the news.
4. Discuss what you should do following the meeting, especially in terms of talking with others; follow these directions.
5. If your supervisor directs you to, consult legal counsel and a malpractice insurance carrier, with your supervisor present.
6. Strongly consider obtaining personal counseling related to the experience, and if you decide against beginning your own counseling, seek out support mechanisms specifically geared toward this sort of event, in order to reduce any sense of isolation you may feel (e.g., books or publications written for survivors, organizations of suicide survivors).
7. Discuss with your supervisor how to inform other staff members and students at the site, and your peer group, as well as your significant others, about the incident. Consider how to obtain support from them.
8. Complete case notes about the news and the supervision session, being careful not to make any self-incriminating or apologetic statements. Be clear about what has been *reported* versus what you know as fact. Do not change or delete entries and do not add predated entries. Such additions to a file could be viewed suspiciously should a clinical review be initiated.
9. Try to obtain facts about the incident from a neutral party, but do not make any statements that may sound like an assumption of responsibility.
10. If your supervisor allows, contact the significant others of the client, but be careful about saying anything that may contribute to anger or guilt among the loved ones or that might lead them to assume negligence on your part.
11. If significant others want to, and your supervisor allows, meet with the family; discuss with your supervisor whether she or he should be present.
12. Consider making a counseling referral for the significant others.

13. Consider whether you want to ask the appropriate person about whether to attend the funeral, wake, or other ritual if death has occurred.
14. Consider whether you would be willing to participate in a psychological autopsy in the future (e.g., 3-6 months later).

Supervisors

1. Follow the training program's/clinic's established policies and procedures related to supervision and students interacting with clients (see below).
2. Rearrange your schedule to allow plenty of time to meet with the supervisee.
3. Allow the supervisee to talk about her or his emotions, thoughts, and fears, without attempting to determine responsibility or judge the adequacy of the supervisee's care.
4. If it seems appropriate, remind the trainee that she or he is not alone in this experience and self-disclose if relevant (note: we say "remind" because we are assuming that training programs and supervisors will have informed supervisees that they are likely to see a client who is suicidal and may have a client attempt or die by suicide, see below).
5. Review the client's file and appropriate portions of relevant audio-/videotapes.
6. Discuss what the supervisee should do and what you will do following the meeting, especially regarding the student talking with others.
7. Discuss with the supervisee whether to cancel any scheduled clients, how to engage in self-care, and consider whether to encourage the student to seek counseling related to the incident. Discuss the grieving process and offer support as the student moves through it.
8. Discuss with the supervisee how to inform other staff members and students at the site, and the student's peer group, as well as her or his significant others, about the incident. Consider how the trainee can obtain support from them.
9. Discuss what sort of record keeping needs to take place.
10. Document the supervision session and recommendations; continue keeping contemporaneous supervision notes as other meetings, interventions, consultations occur related to the incident.
11. Consult your own superiors, legal counsel, and malpractice insurance carrier.
12. If necessary, involve the student in the meetings outlined in #11.
13. Try to obtain facts about the incident from a neutral party, but do not make any statements that may sound like an assumption of responsibility on your part or the trainee's.

14. Consider whether the student should try to contact the significant others of the client. If so, remind her or him to be careful about maintaining the client's confidentiality and about saying anything that may contribute to anger or guilt among the loved ones or that might lead them to assume negligence on the trainee's or your part.
15. Consider whether it would be acceptable to allow the trainee to meet with the client's significant others, if that is what they want; consider whether you want to be present.
16. Suggest the trainee consider making a counseling referral for the significant others.
17. Discuss with the student whether she or he wants to ask the appropriate person about whether to attend the funeral, wake, or other ritual if death has occurred.
18. Discuss with the student whether she or he would be willing to participate in a psychological autopsy in the future (e.g., 3-6 months later).
19. Act as an advocate for the supervisee in situations where it appears as if others may be penalizing or attempting to assign blame to the student, or pressuring the student to "get over" the grief she or he may be feeling.
20. Monitor the supervisee's emotional state; work with clients (especially those who present with depression, suicidality, or somehow resemble the client who attempted or completed suicide); and interactions with peers, faculty, and staff.
21. Monitor your own involvement such that the supervisory relationship with the trainee does not change into a counseling relationship. If you become aware that you are acting as your trainee's counselor, albeit unintentionally, reconsider referring the student for her or his own personal counseling.

Training Programs/Sites

Before an Attempt or Death Occurs

1. Most importantly, administrators must remember that suicide can and does happen in the mental health industry and must keep in mind that despite the best and most professional efforts of even well-trained and experienced therapists and trainees, sometimes a client will attempt or die by suicide.
2. Attempt to foster a supportive, nonjudgmental, and non-blaming atmosphere that allows students to experience and share their concerns and feelings.
3. Ensure that supervisors are well trained in suicide-related issues. Develop written guidelines about the confidential nature of supervisory records and conversations, especially in situations where there has been a suicide attempt or death.

4. Develop a training program for students about suicide assessment and intervention. As part of the training incorporate data on the incidence of suicide attempts and completions experienced by trainees and professionals and the types of sequelae that may follow an attempt or death. Ensure that students are educated about how much control or responsibility they have with clients (especially in outpatient settings) and that there are natural and acceptable limits on what the student can offer (e.g., the student is allowed to go on vacation even if a client is depressed: training must end at some point). Make sure trainees and supervisors are aware of the post-incident protocol (see below).
5. Establish guidelines for meeting with supervisors; obtaining additional consultation; and documenting sessions, supervision, and consultations.
6. Develop an "impossible case" or "person at risk" conference where students can learn about difficult clients and outcomes. Institute nonjudgmental "psychological autopsy" conferences as appropriate. Institute written guidelines about the confidential nature of these sessions, consult with an attorney about how to ensure the information remains privileged in the event of a suit or ethics charge.
7. Contract with a consultant and develop an ongoing support group for students who have experienced a suicide attempt or death.
8. Attempt to assign clients to supervisees based upon skill and experience of the student.
9. Ensure that the site has clients sign paperwork acknowledging that they are seeing a student.
10. Ensure that intake paperwork includes a section asking the client about prior mental health treatment and history of taking psychotropic medications. If the client has a history of either or both, make sure it is standard practice for students to attempt to obtain prior mental health/medical records. Be sure this is documented in the file.

After an Attempt or Death Occurs

1. All faculty/staff should demonstrate empathy, unconditional support, and respect.
2. Have the student and supervisor meet (see above).
3. After the supervisor and trainee meet, the supervisor should meet with her or his superiors to discuss the incident, inform legal counsel, and malpractice insurance carrier. If necessary, include the student in such meetings.
4. As additional information becomes available, revisit plans and needs.
5. Encourage the student to use the confidential impossible case conference or psychological autopsy to allow the student, her or his peers, and faculty/staff to learn from the situation.

6. Do not allow other students, faculty, or staff to penalize, attempt to assign blame, or pressure the student to "get over" the grief she or he may be feeling.
7. Do not attempt to minimize the impact of the incident on the student, peers, supervisor, faculty/staff; determine how the event can be used to help the program and student.
8. Allow the supervisee to grieve.

We believe that following these guidelines will help training programs/sites and supervisors provide appropriate and sufficient support to trainees who experience a client's suicide attempt or death. Although each student's experience and reaction will be different, the literature seems consistent enough to support the outline we have provided. We also hope that our suggestions will help trainees themselves be more aware and prepared if they experience such an event and will help them get the support they need in such a difficult time. We encourage continued exploration into these issues and hope that more discussions will take place in the literature about what trainees experience and how programs have helped them in the wake of a suicide attempt or death.

REFERENCES

Alexander, D. A., Klein, S., Gray, N. M., Dewar, I. G., & Eagles, J. M. (2000). Suicide by patients: Questionnaire study of its effects on consultant psychiatrists. *British Medical Journal, 320,* 1571-1574.

Bongar, B. (2002). *The suicidal patient: Clinical and legal standards of care* (2nd ed.). Washington, DC: American Psychological Association.

Bongar, B., Berman, A. L., Maris, R. W., Silverman, M. M., Harris, E. A., & Packman, W. L. (Eds.). (1998). *Risk management with suicidal patients.* New York: Guilford.

Bongar, B., & Harmatz, M. (1989). Graduate training in clinical psychology and the study of suicide. *Professional Psychology: Research and Practice, 20,* 209-213.

Bongar, B., Maris, R. W., Berman, A. L., & Litman, R. E. (1998). Outpatient standards of care and the suicidal patient. In B. Bongar, A. L. Berman, R. W. Maris, M. M. Silverman, E. A. Harris, & W. L. Packman (Eds.), *Risk management with suicidal patients* (pp. 4-33). New York: Guilford.

Brown, H. N. (1987). The impact of suicide on therapists in training. *Comprehensive Psychiatry, 28,* 101-112.

Brown, H. N. (1989). Patient suicide and therapists in training. In D. Jacobs & H. N. Brown (Eds.), *Suicide: Understanding and responding* (pp. 415-434). Madison, CT: International Universities Press.

Carter, R. E. (1971). Some effects of client suicide on the therapist. *Psychotherapy: Theory, Research and Practice, 8,* 287-289.

Chemtob, C. M., Hamada, R. S., Bauer, G., Kinney, B., & Torigoe, R. Y. (1988). Patients' suicides: Frequency and impact on psychiatrists. *American Journal of Psychiatry, 145,* 224-228.

Chemtob, C. M., Hamada, R. S., Bauer, G., Torigoe, R. Y., & Kinney, B. (1988). Patient suicide: Frequency and impact on psychologists. *Professional Psychology: Research and Practice, 19,* 416-420.

DeAngelis, T. (2001, November). Surviving a patient's suicide. *Monitor on Psychology, 32*(10), 70-73.

Deutsch, C. (1984). Self-reported sources of stress among psychotherapists. *Professional Psychology: Research and Practice, 15,* 833-845.

Ellis, T. E., & Dickey, T. O. (1998). Procedures surrounding the suicide of a trainee's patient: A national survey of psychology internships and psychiatry residency programs. *Professional Psychology: Research and Practice, 29,* 492-497.

Ellis, T. E., & Jones, E. C. (1995, August). *What if my intern's patient commits suicide? Results of a national survey.* Paper presented at the 103rd Annual Convention of the American Psychological Association, New York, NY.

Feldman, D. (1987). A social work student's reaction to client suicide. *Social Casework: The Journal of Contemporary Social Work, 68,* 184-187.

Goldstein, L. S., & Buongiorno, P. A. (1984). Psychotherapists as suicide survivors. *American Journal of Psychotherapy, 38,* 392-397.

Holden, L. D. (1978). Therapist response to patient suicide: Professional and personal. *Journal of Continuing Education in Psychiatry, 39,* 23-32.

Jobes, D. A., & Berman, A. L. (1993). Suicide and malpractice liability: Assessing and revising policies, procedures, and practice in outpatient settings. *Professional Psychology: Research and Practice, 24,* 91-99.

Jobes, D. A., & Maltsberger, J. T. (1995). The hazards of treating suicidal patients. In M. B. Sussman (Ed.), *A perilous calling: The hazards of psychotherapy practice* (pp. 200-214). New York: John Wiley & Sons.

Jones, F. A., Jr. (1987). Therapists as survivors of client suicide. In E. J. Dunne, J. L. McIntosh, & K. Dunne-Maxim (Eds.), *Suicide and its aftermath: Understanding and counseling the survivors* (pp. 126-141). New York: W.W. Norton.

Kaye, N. S., & Soreff, S. M. (1991). The psychiatrist's role, responses, and responsibilities: When a patient commits suicide. *American Journal of Psychiatry, 148,* 739-743.

Kleespies, P. M. (1993). The stress of patient suicidal behavior: Implications for interns and training programs in psychology. *Professional Psychology: Research and Practice, 24,* 477-482.

Kleespies, P. M., Niles, B. L., Mori, D. L., & Deleppo, J. D. (1998). Emergencies with suicidal patients: The impact on the clinician. In P. M. Kleespies (Ed.), *Emergencies in mental health practice: Evaluation and management* (pp. 379-397). New York: Guilford.

Kleespies, P. M., Penk, W. E., & Forsyth, J. P. (1993). The stress of patient suicidal behavior during clinical training: Incidence, impact, and recovery. *Professional Psychology: Research and Practice, 24,* 293-303.

Kleespies, P. M., Smith, M. R., & Becker, B. R. (1990). Psychology interns as patient suicide survivors: Incidence, impact, and recovery. *Professional Psychology: Research and Practice, 21,* 257-263.

Kolodny, S., Binder, R. L., Bronstein, A. A., & Friend, R. L. (1979). The working through of patients' suicides by four therapists. *Suicide and Life-Threatening Behavior, 9,* 33-46.

Kozlowska, S., Nunn, K., & Cousens, P. (1997). Training in psychiatry: An examination of trainee perceptions. Part I. *Australian and New Zealand Journal of Psychiatry, 31,* 641-652.

Litman, R. E. (1965). When patients commit suicide. *American Journal of Psychotherapy, 19,* 570-576.

Lynch, V. J. (1987). Supervising the trainee who treats the chronically suicidal outpatient: Theoretical perspectives and practice approaches. *The Clinical Supervisor, 5,* 99-110.

Marshall, K. A. (1980). When a patient commits suicide. *Suicide and Life-Threatening Behavior, 10,* 29-39.

Menninger, W. W. (1991). Patient suicide and its impact on the psychotherapist. *Bulletin of the Menninger Clinic, 55,* 216-227.

Packman, W. L., & Harris, E. A. (1998). Legal issues and risk management in suicidal patients. In B. Bongar, A. L. Berman, R. W. Maris, M. M. Silverman, E. A. Harris, & W. L. Packman (Eds.), *Risk management with suicidal patients* (pp. 150-186). New York: Guilford.

Ruben, H. L. (1990). Surviving a suicide in your practice. In S. J. Blumenthal & D. J. Kupfer (Eds.), *Suicide over the life cycle: Risk factors, assessment, and treatment of suicidal patients* (pp. 619-636). Washington, DC: American Psychiatric Press.

Shein, H. M. (1976). Suicide care: Obstacles in the education of psychiatric residents. *Omega, 7,* 75-81.

Spiegelman, J. S. (2001, January/February). Losing a client to suicide: The experience of a new clinician. *The Los Angeles Psychologist,* 12-13.

Spiegelman, J. S., Ellis, T. E., Briggs, M. L., & Rogers, J. R. (2000). Supervisory issues around client suicides. In M. Weishaar (Ed.), *Suicide '99: Proceedings of the 32nd Annual Conference of the American Association of Suicidology* (pp. 99-100). Washington, DC: American Association of Suicidology.

Spiegelman, J. S., & Rogers, J. R. (2000). Suicide and supervision: Postvention with trainees. In M. Weishaar (Ed.), *Suicide '99 Proceedings of the 32nd Annual Conference of the American Association of Suicidology* (pp. 101-102). Washington, DC: American Association of Suicidology.

Tanney, B. (1995). After a suicide: A helper's handbook. In B. L. Mishara (Ed.), *The impact of suicide* (pp. 100-120). New York: Springer.

Valente, S. (1994). Psychotherapist reactions to the suicide of a patient. *American Journal of Orthopsychiatry, 64,* 614-621.

Werth, J. L., Jr., Burke, C., & Bardash, R. J. (2002). Confidentiality in end-of-life and after-death situations. *Ethics and Behavior, 12,* 205-222.

Suggestions for Supervisors
When a Therapist Experiences
a Client's Suicide

Doreen Schultz

SUMMARY. The suicide of a client can have a profound effect on both the therapist and the supervisory relationship. This paper addresses some of the known reactions to client suicide and clinical themes as noted in the literature and in the experiences of several therapists. It also provides some beginning considerations and suggestions for the supervisory relationship, as well as notes some directions for research in this area. *[Article copies available for a fee from The Haworth Document Delivery Service: 1-800-HAWORTH. E-mail address: <docdelivery@haworthpress.com> Website: <http://www.HaworthPress.com> © 2005 by The Haworth Press, Inc. All rights reserved.]*

KEYWORDS. Client suicide, suicide, supervision

Doreen Schultz, MA NCC, is a doctoral student in Counseling Psychology at Georgia State University. She is also the Associate Director for The Link's National Resource Center for Suicide Prevention and Aftercare, Atlanta, GA.

Address correspondence to: Doreen Schultz, Georgia State University, College of Education, Department of Counseling and Psychological Services, Atlanta, GA 30303.

[Haworth co-indexing entry note]: "Suggestions for Supervisors When a Therapist Experiences a Client's Suicide." Schultz, Doreen. Co-published simultaneously in *Women & Therapy* (The Haworth Press, Inc.) Vol. 28, No. 1, 2005, pp. 59-69; and: *Therapeutic and Legal Issues for Therapists Who Have Survived a Client Suicide: Breaking the Silence* (ed: Kayla Miriyam Weiner) The Haworth Press, Inc., 2005, pp. 59-69. Single or multiple copies of this article are available for a fee from The Haworth Document Delivery Service [1-800-HAWORTH, 9:00 a.m. - 5:00 p.m. (EST). E-mail address: docdelivery@haworthpress.com].

http://www.haworthpress.com/web/WT
© 2005 by The Haworth Press, Inc. All rights reserved.
Digital Object Identifier: 10.1300/J015v28n01_05

The death of a patient by suicide has been called "the ultimate peril for the psychotherapist" (Jobes & Maltsberger, 1995, p. 200). For the therapist that has had a client die by suicide, the grief experience can be arduous and complicated. The suicide of a client can also pose a unique challenge for the supervisor working with the therapist-survivor in addressing both the professional issues as well as the therapist's feelings of trauma and grief. This article describes some of the reactions experienced by therapist-survivors of suicide, notes some of the implications and suggestions for the supervisory relationship, and offers some directions for future research. While reference to legal implications is made, the suggestions here are intended for situations where no clinical negligence has been found, and are grounded in the existing research and experience of many therapists.

THERAPISTS AS SURVIVORS:
PERSONAL AND PROFESSIONAL REACTIONS

In his review of the literature, Jones (1987) noted that therapists have both personal and professional reactions to client suicide. Personal reactions may span the full range of emotions and may be complicated by individual factors, such as the therapist's own bereavement history and personal experience with suicide. Personal reactions to client suicide may also be affected by the therapist's previous experience with other traumatic events. One therapist-survivor indicated that following a client's suicide he was having nightmares of an armed robbery he had witnessed several years earlier. Clinicians with a personal history of trauma may find that their client's suicide reawakens feelings related to past trauma, whether suicide-related or not. Horn's (1994) review of the literature suggests that other factors may affect the therapist's reaction to a client's suicide, including life experiences, work involvement, and the therapist's own beliefs about his or her role as a helping professional.

Professional reactions may also include fears of blame from the family, censure by colleagues and doubts regarding competence (Jones, 1987). Therapist-survivors may feel the professional stigma of suicide, believing that others see the suicide of their client as evidence that they mismanaged the case (Jobes & Maltsberger, 1995).

INDIVIDUAL FACTORS RELATED TO THE THERAPY
AND THE SUICIDE

A therapist's reaction to the suicide of a client may also be affected by individual circumstances related to the therapy and the suicide. While each therapeutic experience is unique, how the therapist learned of the suicide and whether the client made reference to the therapy at the time of her or his death are two examples of circumstances that may affect the therapist's response.

How the therapist learns of the suicide may be crucial to understanding how she or he may react. One therapist informed me that she became aware of the suicide of a former client by seeing the obituary in the paper a year after the client had ended therapy. Another mental health professional who worked in a residential treatment facility learned of a client's suicide on site, after discovering the client's body. Each of these therapists grieved their client's suicide, but their reactions were quite different. The therapist reading the obituary a year later indicated feeling mostly sadness but little professional responsibility, given that the client had not indicated suicidality during the therapy. The mental health professional that discovered his client's suicide on site experienced a significant level of trauma related to the scene he witnessed, as well as anger toward the client for exposing other clients in the facility to the trauma of the client's suicide.

Whether the client referred to the therapy near the time of her or his death may also affect the therapist's reaction to the death. For example, one clinician received a telephone message from her client indicating that he was unhappy with the progress of the therapy and would not be continuing. He did not respond to her telephone calls requesting him to come in for a final session and was found dead several days later from a self-inflicted gunshot wound. For this therapist, this last message from her client affected her for years following the suicide. In another case, a therapist received a suicide note from her client written at the time of his death, apologizing to the therapist for the act and for not being honest with her in the therapy. She noted that knowing that the client had not told her everything relieved some of her feelings of responsibility about what she could have done to help the client. Both of these therapists will grieve their client's death, but the supervisor working with each of them will need to be aware of how these differences could affect their grief response.

Another variable that may have an impact on how a therapist-survivor reacts to a client's suicide is the therapist's gender. Grad, Zavasnik, and Groleger (1997) found in their study that women therapists felt shame and guilt and doubted their professional knowledge more often than their male counterparts. Women were also more likely to seek consolation from others following the suicide of their client than were men. More men reported returning to work as usual following the suicide than women (Grad et al., 1997). Gender differences can also provide information for the supervisor who is trying to best support her or his supervisee at this critical time.

IMPLICATIONS FOR THE SUPERVISORY RELATIONSHIP

The experience of client suicide has a profound and often lasting effect on the therapist, both personally and professionally. Therapists often need support in grieving this loss both from other professionals and from the therapist's own personal support network. Support is crucial to the healing of both the personal and professional wounds following a suicide. Hendlin, Lipschitz, Maltsberger, Haas, and Wynecoop (2000) noted that therapist-survivors reported feeling less isolated when colleagues and supervisors offered support by sharing their own experiences with client suicide, and found this more helpful than reassurances related to the treatment process.

Unfortunately, therapist-survivors are often left to find their own comfort and receive little support from the institutional review of the cases (Hendlin et al., 2000). Sadly, therapists may make decisions about their professional competence when this support is lacking, despite no evidence of clinical wrongdoing. One colleague decided to leave the profession following the suicide of her client in a residential facility in which she worked due to the lack of support from the institution. Lack of support, whether real or imagined, may contribute to the therapist survivors' feelings of isolation and guilt.

Despite the importance of the supervisor's role following a suicide, the therapist-survivor may not seek support from the supervisor following a suicide, perhaps out of fear of being blamed for the suicide. In Grad et al. (1997), less than half of the therapist-survivor participants indicated that they spoke with their supervisor about the suicide, though more than half indicated that talking to others had helped them the most.

In many settings supervisors are charged with the duty of participating in a formal case review as well as providing support for the bereaved therapist. The supervisor can expect to be part of a formal and informal review of the case with the therapist. Often, the formal review is done as part of the institutional review process following a client's death. While the formal case review can help both the therapist and the supervisor process the client suicide, the therapist may also see it as a critical process. For this reason, Gorkin (1985) has suggested that formal reviews to determine negligence occur separately from informal reviews (as cited in Jones, 1987). This is with the intention to help the therapist to process the feelings related to the suicide. Stelovich (1999) offered some suggestions for conducting a suicide review, though each system may have its own unique requirements. Even if no negligence is found in a formal review, legal proceedings initiated by the client's family may still occur. Supervision and consultation, as well as full reviews of case consultation notes, often help the therapist against charges of negligence (Jobes & Maltsberger, 1995). If wrongly accused of negligence, the supervisor needs to advocate for the therapist as well as be aware of system policies and procedures that can be of assistance.

If no negligence is found, the supervisor still has the responsibility to assist the therapist in working through the professional and personal issues following the suicide. Dunne (1987a) noted that suicide survivors have special needs in therapy. Given the challenges of losing a client to suicide, it is assumed that they also have special needs in supervision. Dunne labeled several clinical themes that occur in therapy with suicide survivors. These themes are used here to describe some of the potential implications for supervision with therapist-survivors. Dunne noted that these themes are not meant to describe the survivor as much as to serve as reminders of the unique issues that will arise following a suicide. Again, how these themes play a role in the supervisory interaction will also depend on the individual factors. Dunne's (1987a) clinical themes and their implications for clinical supervision follow below.

1. The survivor's perpetual need to search for both physical and psychological cues as to the reason of the suicide. (Dunne, 1987a)

The search for "why" is an important part of healing for any survivor of suicide. The search for physical and psychological cues may involve detailed reviews of the case over several supervision sessions, where the therapist explores different aspects of the therapeutic relationship in search of cues that may have indicated the possibility of suicide. It may also involve the therapist searching for evidence outside of the therapeutic relationship, such as talking to the client's family, or reviewing events just before the client's death. Dunne (1987a) notes that for the survivor, this search for answers is an ongoing attempt to obtain closure on this painful experience.

The supervisor needs to allow the therapist time to explore the "why" in supervision. Because this may take the time of other tasks of the supervision, the supervisor may find that additional supervision time is needed. Additionally, the clinical supervisor should be aware of whether the search for "why" is having negative consequences. Berman (1995) gives a good example of a therapist that sent a letter to the client's family following the client's death. The letter, written out the therapist's desire to help the family but also to defend himself, was met with anger and resentment from the client's family. Such experiences need to be attended to throughout the clinical supervision, as they may exacerbate feelings of guilt and responsibility.

2. Whether irrational or appropriate, surviving suicide leaves a legacy of inexorable guilt. (Dunne, 1987a, p. 201)

Feelings of guilt are a normal experience following a suicide, and a survivor may revisit several aspects of their relationship with the deceased in an attempt to relieve her or his feelings of guilt. A therapist's guilt may arise from feelings of what the therapist may have done differently in the therapy having the knowledge that the client would die by suicide. Hendlin et al. (2000) noted that the majority of therapists in their study identified at least one change they would have made in their clients' treatment. Looking for ways to improve services can be an important and positive outcome of this tragedy. However, supervisors may find that supervisees may have an unrealistic idea of what they could have done differently, affected by knowledge they may not have had prior to the suicide and feelings of guilt. Supervisors may remind supervisees that even if they had done things differently in the treatment, there are no guarantees that the outcome of suicide would have been different.

Supervisors should also be wary of urges to rescue the therapist from these feelings of guilt. Whether irrational or not, survivors of suicide often feel guilt as a normal response to suicide, and avoidance of these feelings can lead to complications later in the grief process. On the other hand, some therapists may not avoid feelings of guilt but immerse themselves in them. Therapists may also look to eradicate feelings of guilt by approaching the deceased family and claiming some responsibility for the suicide. Gutheil (1999) noted that the literature suggests that neither immersion in guilt or avoidance of it is helpful. He recommended that regrets should be shared with supervisors or peers instead of the client's family. Instead, if the therapist chooses to approach the family, she or he should do so expressing remembrance of positive qualities of the deceased, as families are often struggling with acknowledging the positive in light of the tragedy (Gutheil, 1999). Supervisors may need to explore with their supervisees their plans to approach the family and how their feelings of guilt or responsibility may affect these interactions. Additionally, the supervisor may help the therapist in making referrals to the family for support services following the suicide, if appropriate.

> 3. Social relationships are altered following a suicide as a consequence of real or imagined stigma. (Dunne, 1987a)

Survivors of suicide often report changes in social relationships due to the stigma of losing a loved one to suicide. While this may also be true for the therapist who loses a client to suicide, it can be very significant if those changes occur with work colleagues from whom the therapist derives support. Hopefully, the therapist-survivor is met with support from colleagues. Unfortunately, sometimes therapist-survivors encounter unhelpful responses from their colleagues, which contribute to feelings of stigma. More often colleagues may avoid the therapist-survivor, ignoring the event. This, too, can contribute to the feelings of stigma. Supporters may also experience a survivor syndrome, or relief that it was not their client who ended his or her life (Tanney, 1995).

The role of the supervisor, particularly in a setting where many are likely to know about the suicide, is to encourage the expression of support for the therapist. This includes taking an active stance in squelching rumors related to the suicide or the therapy. This is best achieved by providing information to the staff that is clear, accurate and timely (Dunne, 1987b). It also involves being an advocate for the therapist when administrative procedures exist that may contribute to feelings of stigma. In one situation, an administrative decision was made to prohibit a therapist-survivor from seeing new clients for an extended period, despite no negligence found on the part of the therapist. The decision was made with the good intention of giving the therapist time to work through her feelings about the suicide, which she was doing in her own personal therapy and in supervision. Because the intention was not clearly communicated to the therapist, she reported feeling the stigma of suicide each hour she was not allowed to see a new client while her colleagues had full schedules. The role of the supervisor is also to advocate for clear communication to the therapist regarding administrative procedures as well as to encourage supportive social relationships.

4. Grief following a suicide is complex and likely to be incomplete. (Dunne, 1987a)

Therapist-survivors may experience a complex grief reaction to a client's suicide that resembles symptoms of Posttraumatic Stress Disorder (PTSD). A complex grief reaction following suicide may involve intrusive symptoms, such as nightmares or flashbacks related to the client's suicide as well as numbing and avoidance of reminders of the event. For the therapist, these symptoms may manifest by an increase in time away from the office. Cleiren and Diekstra (1995) noted that strong posttraumatic stress reactions as an early reaction to the loss may be a strong indication of future problems in adaptation. Traumatic responses are a complex part of suicide bereavement to which the therapist is not immune.

The grief following suicide is often incomplete because of the many unanswered questions and difficulty achieving closure on the loss. For the therapist-survivor this may be exacerbated by an inability to participate in rituals that may be healing, such as spending time with others that were close to the client. Additionally, therapist-survivors may notice upsurges of grief related to the suicide, as grieving a suicide is generally a nonlinear process (Dunne, 1987a). These upsurges can be triggered by a number of things, including the anniversary of the client's death or other losses that the therapist may experience.

The supervisor may also assist the therapist by providing education on how grief responses may manifest some time after the suicide. Special care should be taken to explore what options are available to the therapist if he or she is experiencing a complicated grief response, including reducing workload or taking personal time if requested by the therapist. The supervisor may also need to meet with the therapist more frequently on an "as-needed" basis when the therapist is experiencing an upsurge of grief. The supervisor will also need to be aware of any residual grief issues that impede the therapist's ability to work with other clients and address them as appropriate. This may involve a referral to therapy or support groups for survivors of suicide.

5. The idea of suicide as a solution to a problem becomes implanted in the mind of the survivor. (Dunne, 1987a, p. 204)

In Berman (1995), a therapist-survivor described it this way: "My philosophy has changed. I now consider all of my patients suicidal as well as myself" (p. 97). For the therapist-survivor, this clinical theme of suicide as a solution may develop in two ways. First, the clinical supervisor may notice that the therapist-survivor is assessing for suicide more frequently in more clients. This may be, in part, due to the therapist's realization that many consider suicide as a solution to a problem. In Hendlin et al. (2000), all of the therapist-survivor participants noted being more alert to the possibility of suicide in their clients.

The second way this theme may manifest in therapist-survivors is in their own thoughts of suicide. Unfortunately, therapists do end their lives. A client's suicide may exacerbate existing distress in therapists who are experiencing personal crises. The American Counseling Association noted that supervisors are responsible for recognizing personal impairment that would affect the supervisee's ability to perform competent clinical services (as cited in Falvey, 2002). Haas and Hall (1991) recommended that the supervisor provide close supervision of the therapist's activities and may need to impose limits on professional activities if impairment becomes an issue (as cited in Falvey, 2002). It is important that the supervisor balances their professional responsibilities with sensitivity in helping the therapist work through her or his distress.

6. Suicide affects the capacity to trust others. (Dunne, 1987a)

In experiencing a client's suicide, therapist-survivors may have difficulty trusting other clients. In many cases, the client may have told the therapist that she or he would not harm her- or himself. Therapists may also have had their clients sign "no-harm" contracts prior to the suicide. The therapist-survivor may have difficulty trusting other clients in similar situations or may have a general feeling of mistrust about what clients say in session. Therapist-survivors may find that they are having more difficulty trusting their own clinical judgment and client conceptualizations. Losing trust in both clients and their ability to help them deeply affects therapists' feelings of competence as helping professionals. Brown (1987) noted that more experienced therapists are often better able to see a client's suicide as part of the limitations of therapy as opposed to their own incompetence. However, Hendlin et al. (2000) noted that even veteran therapists in their study were surprised to learn that a client's suicide affected their level of self-doubt. Therapists in training also questioned their skills as helping professionals and how suited they were for the profession (Hendlin et al., 2000).

The supervisor can help the therapist-survivor regain trust in her or his abilities as a therapist by helping connect the survivor with other therapists who have lost clients to suicide. If the supervisor has had such an experience, sharing that with the therapist can have a profound effect on the therapist's perceptions about professional competence. Despite the fact that many therapists have had clients die by suicide, many do not openly share this information. This adds to the perception of the therapist-survivor that this is an extremely rare event. Learning that other competent professionals have had clients die by suicide can go far in helping the therapist regain a sense of trust in her or his abilities and the profession.

The therapist-survivor may also benefit from a candid discussion in supervision about how the suicide has changed the therapist's clinical work and focus. It is difficult to imagine an experience shaking one's foundations of trust and not being changed by it both personally and professionally. Some therapists may find a calling toward working with suicidal patients or those bereaved by suicide. Others may find that they approach their clients with a new level of sensitivity not known before the suicide. Recognizing both the tragedy, as well as any positive changes that have occurred following the suicide, can help the therapist integrate the experience into her or his life. This may help the therapist see the client's suicide as an experience that helped strengthen her or his professional work rather than diminish it.

FINAL CONSIDERATIONS AND SUGGESTIONS FOR RESEARCH

Foster and McAdams (1999) reminded us that it is the responsibility of the supervisor to initiate a response to client suicide rather than rely on the supervisees' initiative. Particularly for supervisees' early in their career, this point needs to be underscored. Additionally, the supervisor may benefit from consultation with colleagues or other professionals when providing assistance following a client suicide (Foster & McAdams, 1999). The supervisor is not expected to know it all, and can be most effective when she or he realizes that the more information made available to the therapist-survivor the more likely will be the healing. While training programs specifically in suicidology are scarce, resources exist to help therapists learn more about suicide. Recently, a therapist-survivor task force was formed by the American Association of Suicidology (AAS) as a resource to therapists and other interested individuals (AAS, 2001). Other groups, such as The Link's National Resource Center for Suicide Prevention and Aftercare in Atlanta, Georgia, provide consultation to professionals and others following a suicide.

Supervisors in some settings may find that they have teams of professionals who have been traumatized by a client suicide. Critical Incident Stress Debriefing (CISD) (Mitchell & Everly, 1993) is one model that has been adapted for survivors of suicide (Juhnke & Shoffner, 1999). While such models are not meant to substitute for supervision or other professional support, they can be an effective initial intervention with mental health providers surviving the suicide of a client. A combination of early intervention, continued supervision, ongoing personal and professional support, and connection to further resources seem to be the best tools in helping therapist-survivors work through the trauma of client suicide.

McIntosh (1987) provided an important overview of the literature regarding research with suicide survivors. He noted that longitudinal and follow-up investigations have generally been missing from survivor research, and retrospective studies have dominated the existing research (McIntosh, 1987). McAdams and Foster (2000) noted that research specific to therapist-survivors has focused mainly on the disciplines of psychiatry and psychology. Additional research is needed to assess the problem of client suicide in other disciplines, such as social work and counseling (Foster & McAdams, 1999). Additionally, studies with larger samples using non-report measures would yield more generalizable results with greater reliability (Foster & McAdams, 1999).

Research that considers variables such as age, race, circumstances of the suicide and practice settings would provide more information about how these factors might influence therapist's response (Foster & McAdams, 1999). More qualitative studies that follow the Suicide Data Bank project (Hendlin et al., 2000) would provide valuable information as to some of the responses and problems faced by therapists following the suicide of a client. Research concerning supervisor's responses to therapist-survivors will also provide information about best practices in supervision following a suicide. Research concerning public perceptions of therapist-survivors may help us to better understand the origins of stigma. Finally, studies that evaluate interventions with therapist-survivors, such as support groups, individual therapy, and stress-debriefing models, would also yield more information for postvention efforts.

Cantor (1999) expressed the opinion that the problem of suicide may never be eradicated. Whether one agrees with this or not, the supervisor has a responsibility to become more informed about the effects and implications of client suicide for the therapist and the supervisory relationship.

REFERENCES

American Association of Suicidology (2001). *Therapists as survivors of a patient suicide.* [Online]. Available: http://www.suicidology.org/index.html

Berman, A.L. (1995). "To engrave herself on all our memories, to force her body into our lives": The impact of suicide on psychotherapists. In B.L. Mishara (Ed.), *The impact of suicide* (pp. 85-99). New York: Springer.

Brown, H.N. (1987). The impact of client suicide on therapists in training. *Comprehensive Psychiatry, 28(2),* 101-112.

Cantor, P. (1999). Can suicide ever be eradicated? A professional journey. In D.G. Jacobs (Ed.), *The Harvard Medical School guide to suicide assessment and intervention* (pp. 239-248). San Francisco: Jossey-Bass.

Cleiren, M.P. & Diekstra, R.F (1995). After the loss: Bereavement after suicide and other types of death. In B.L. Mishara (Ed.), *The impact of suicide* (pp. 7-39). New York: Springer.

Dunne, E.J. (1987a). Special needs of suicide survivors in therapy. In E.J. Dunne, J.L. McIntosh, & K. Dunne-Maxim (Eds.), *Suicide and its aftermath* (pp. 193-207). New York: Norton & Co.

Dunne, E.J. (1987b). A response to suicide in the mental health setting. In E.J. Dunne, J.L. McIntosh, & K. Dunne-Maxim (Eds.), *Suicide and its aftermath* (pp. 182-192). New York: Norton & Co.

Falvey, J.E. (2002). *Managing clinical supervision: Ethical practice and legal risk management.* Pacific Grove, CA: Brooks/Cole.

Foster, V.A. & Adams, C.R. (1999). The impact of client suicide in counselor training: Implications for counselor education and supervision. *Counselor Education and Supervision, 39(1),* 22-34.

Grad, O.T., Zavasnik, A., and Groleger, U. (1997). Suicide of a patient: Gender differences in bereavement reactions of therapists. *Suicide and Life-Threatening Behavior, 27(4),* 379-386.

Gutheil, T.G. (1999). Liability issues and liability prevention in suicide. In D.G. Jacobs (Ed.), *The Harvard Medical School guide to suicide assessment and intervention* (pp. 561-578). San Francisco: Jossey-Bass.

Hendlin, H., Lipschitz, A., Maltsberger, J.T., Haas, A.P., & Wynecoop, S. (2000). Therapists' reactions to the suicide of a patient. *American Journal of Psychiatry, 157(12),* 2022-2027.

Horn, P.J. (1994). Therapists' psychological adaptation to client suicide. *Psychotherapy, 31(1),* 190-195.

Jobes, D.A. & Maltsberger, J.T. (1995). The hazards of treating suicidal patients. In M.B. Sussman (Ed.), *A perilous calling: The hazards of psychotherapy practice* (pp. 200-216). New York: Wiley & Sons.

Jones, F.A. (1987). Therapists as survivors of client suicide. In E.J. Dunne, J.L. McIntosh, & K. Dunne-Maxim (Eds.), *Suicide and its aftermath* (pp. 126-141). New York: Norton & Co.

Juhnke, G.A. & Shoffner, M.F. (1999). The family debriefing model: An adapted critical incident stress debriefing for parents and older sibling suicide survivors. *Family Journal, 7(4),* 342-348.

McAdams, C.R. & Foster, V.A. (2000). Client suicide: Its frequency and impact on counselors. *Journal of Mental Health Counseling, 22(2),* 107-121.

McIntosh, J.L. (1987). Research, therapy and educational needs. In E.J. Dunne, J.L. McIntosh, & K. Dunne-Maxim (Eds.), *Suicide and its aftermath* (pp. 263-280). New York: Norton & Co.

Mitchell, J.T. & and Everly, G.S. (1993). *Critical Incident Stress Debriefing (CISD): An operations manual for the prevention of traumatic stress among emergency services and disaster workers.* Ellicott City, MD: Chevron.

Stelovich, S. (1999). Guidelines for conducting a suicide review. In D.G. Jacobs (Ed.), *The Harvard Medical School guide to suicide assessment and intervention* (pp. 482-490). San Francisco: Jossey-Bass.

Tanney, B. (1995). After a suicide: A helper's handbook. In B.L. Mishara (Ed.), *The impact of suicide* (pp. 100-122). New York: Springer.

Therapists as Client Suicide Survivors

Onja T. Grad
Konrad Michel

SUMMARY. The paper presents a discussion between two therapists–
one female, the other male, one a clinical psychologist and the other a
psychiatrist, one working in an institution and the other in a private
practice–each surviving the suicide of a client. It discusses what helped

Onja T. Grad, PhD, works at the University Psychiatric Hospital in Slovenia as a
psychotherapist and supervisor in family therapy with the bereaved, especially after
suicide. She organized the first Slovenian crisis line in 1980 and has been working with
suicide survivors since 1989. She is the first recipient of the Farberow Award (1997),
given by the International Association of Suicide Prevention (IASP), for recognition of
her work in the field of bereavement after suicide. She teaches at the Medical School
University of Ljubljana. She published articles and chapters on suicide survivors, held
workshops and led the organizing team for the 8th European symposium on suicide in
2000. She is serving the second mandate as a vice president of IASP. Currently she is
also involved in launching the national program for suicide prevention in Slovenia.

Konrad Michel, MD, PhD, is a psychiatrist and psychotherapist at the University Psychiatric Hospital in Berne, Switzerland, and is in private practice. He also teaches at the
Medical School of Berne. His main research interests are in the doctor-patient relationship with suicidal patients and in different aspects of suicide prevention, such as prevention focused in a primary care setting to prevent hospitalization. He is also working with
the media to develop ways of giving solid, nonsensational information about suicide.

Address correspondence to: Onja T. Grad, University Psychiatric Hospital, Zaloska
29, SI - 1000 Ljubljana, Slovenia, or Konrad Michel (Universitäre Psychiatrische
Dienste (UPD), Murtenstrasse 21, CH-3010 Bern, Switzerland.

[Haworth co-indexing entry note]: "Therapists as Client Suicide Survivors." Grad, Onja T., and Konrad
Michel. Co-published simultaneously in *Women & Therapy* (The Haworth Press, Inc.) Vol. 28, No. 1, 2005,
pp. 71-81; and: *Therapeutic and Legal Issues for Therapists Who Have Survived a Client Suicide: Breaking
the Silence* (ed: Kayla Miriyam Weiner) The Haworth Press, Inc., 2005, pp. 71-81. Single or multiple copies
of this article are available for a fee from The Haworth Document Delivery Service [1-800-HAWORTH, 9:00
a.m. - 5:00 p.m. (EST). E-mail address: docdelivery@haworthpress.com].

http://www.haworthpress.com/web/WT
Digital Object Identifier: 10.1300/J015v28n01_06

them to continue their psychotherapeutic work following the personal trauma. *[Article copies available for a fee from The Haworth Document Delivery Service: 1-800-HAWORTH. E-mail address: <docdelivery@haworthpress. com> Website: <http://www.HaworthPress.com> © 2005 by The Haworth Press, Inc. All rights reserved.]*

KEYWORDS. Suicide, bereavement, therapist's reactions, gender issues

INTRODUCTION

Starting psychotherapy with a new patient is like starting a journey full of uncertainties and obstacles. The initial assessment and diagnosis may give some clues about the prognosis of the disorder and about possible difficulties and risk in psychotherapeutic treatment. However, psychotherapy is not always beneficial for the patient. In spite of an ongoing therapy the patient's mental condition may worsen, sometimes due to reasons that lie outside the psychotherapeutic situation, sometimes due to difficulties that a therapist and a patient encounter in the course of therapy. Therapists may find plausible explanations for negative outcomes, such as lack of motivation on the patient's side, problems with resistance, or a diagnosis of a so-called treatment resistant personality disorder. Everything, however, seems quite different when a patient commits suicide while still in therapy or immediately after ending the therapy relationship.

Suicide of a patient provokes not only professional questions, doubts and explanations, but also personal, basic human feelings, not entirely different from those experienced of the relatives and friends of the deceased. Many people who have experienced a suicide of a patient will agree that the event is etched in the memory as the one of the most traumatic and painful experiences of a professional career. Brown (1987) says, "... with some obvious exaggeration, there are two kinds of psychiatrists: those who have had a patient commit suicide and those that will" (p. 202). Because it usually strikes one unprepared (30% of therapists experience it in their training or at the beginning of their therapeutic work), it is often more difficult to accommodate (Faberow, 2001).

The reactions of therapists range from a total denial and suppression of any emotions to very personal grief reactions, ranging from a shock and disbelief to anger, guilt, shame and devaluation of one's own professional knowledge (Valente, 1994). How a therapist responds to his/her patient's suicide depends on many (unforeseeable) factors. First and most important is his or her own personality and, as a result, a very individual, personal way of dealing with stress, loss and crisis. Another important factor is the therapist's gender that might create some socially expected/required ways of dealing with a problem for men and women. (Grad, Zavasnik & Groleger, 1997). The third factor is the vocation of the therapist, that brings into the therapy process a variety of knowledge, amount of responsibility (if working in a team), style of approaching the problem and distancing from it, social expectations, ways of communicating about the traumatic experience, and ways of coping. The fourth, but not least important, seems to be one's experiences acquired throughout the working years as a therapist: how one views their status in a hierarchy, the connection of the event to other life experiences, the wisdom and acceptance of limitations by the individual (Alexander et al., 2000; Grad, 1996). The fifth factor is rather plain but yet quite important–the fear of legal litigation.

Depending on the factors mentioned above, there is a question of what help is needed by the therapist after his/her patient has completed suicide. Help should be personalized and individualized to the needs of the particular therapist, while a basic protocol should have been prepared in advance.

CASE VIGNETTES

We will try to show differences in therapist's response based on the factors listed above with four short case presentations treated by two therapists: first a female and then a male; the former a clinical psychologist and the latter a psychiatrist; outpatient and inpatient settings; when the same therapist was still in training and when she/he had become an experienced therapist; when a therapist was backed up by the institution and when she/he was in a private setting.

A. The therapist: A clinical psychologist, female, age 26, second year of residency, work setting: mental health institution

Jane was a 24-year-old teacher, married for two years to an artist–a painter, without children, with a history of depression, treated by a psychiatrist on an outpatient basis for two years. During these two years she was hospitalized once on the ward for psychiatric crisis intervention, diagnosed as "depressed state in neurotic personality," treated with antidepressants and psychotherapy, discharged with no medications and referred to the resident in clinical psychology for outpatient psychotherapy. The patient and therapist began working together very enthusiastically. For the first two months Jane came twice a week and then later once a week for a total of thirteen months. The therapist had regular supervision with a senior colleague throughout therapy. The patient's problems were identified as quarreling with her husband, difficulty separating from her parents, and career ambivalence. These issues were discussed and seemed to result in partial progress; she became more independent, more self-confident and self-satisfied, she even decided to start her master's degree program. Slowly the depressive mood started crawling in, inhibiting her plans. More and more sessions were full of crying and self-accusation, and both the supervisor and therapist felt that more than outpatient psychotherapy was needed. A psychiatrist was consulted for medication, and it was decided to keep Jane in outpatient treatment. However, the antidepressants didn't help, her mood deteriorated, and the therapist (working at the ward for crisis intervention) proposed hospitalization. Jane was very reluctant and wanted to stay with the therapist on a more frequent basis. This was tried again with no success, and in the next session the therapist insisted that she stay on the ward. The patient reluctantly agreed but wanted to go home to get some personal items and promised to come back the same day. She was permitted to go home, but instead of coming back to the hospital, she parked her car at the railway and threw herself in front of the train.

B. The therapist: A clinical psychologist, female, aged 40, 14 years of practice, work setting: mental health institution

Andrea was a 21-year-old student, hospitalized on the crisis intervention unit for extremely aggressive reactions towards a girl she thought was interfering with her boyfriend. She had earlier broken her opponent's hand. She became very withdrawn, insecure, started to spend more and more nights by her mother's bed and didn't want to socialize any more. Previously she had gone to England with her boyfriend and stayed there for a year, working and taking care of herself. The parents were quite upset with her current behavior. They had some marital problems of their own and had been talking of a permanent separation or possibly divorce. Andrea was an only child, always rebellious and difficult, yet very attached to both parents. Her disturbed behavior served to keep her parents together in a mutual caretaking of her. The divorce threat was dropped for the time being when Andrea became so disturbed. While on the ward Andrea became very constructive, pleasant, and took care of other patients. Her behavior was adapted and placid. While in the hospital she found herself a temporary job for the time after her release and made plans to return to school the next academic year. Before the discharge from the hospital the whole family gathered and decided they would make an effort to deal with their problems together in a systemic family therapy setting on an outpatient basis. The working hypothesis was that the patient's regression served the system not to disintegrate, so the final goal of the therapy should be that Andrea stop taking care of her parents' well-being and work through her separation from them. Two family therapists (a clinical psychologist and a psychiatrist) were appointed to start therapy with this family. They worked with them with limited success, when Andrea, after fierce fights with her parents, disclosed her father's many love affairs. After doing so, she became anxious and on the edge of psychosis. She was admitted to the hospital, prescribed medication, and family therapy was proceeding while she was hospitalized. She was angry, threatened suicide very openly and (as wrongly assessed) seemed manipulative and provocative: "I'll go and kill myself and you'll regret it as hell." After a morning group therapy session on the ward, where she was active and didn't seem to be depressed or worried, she went to the castle tower in the middle of the town and threw herself off.

C. The therapist: A psychiatrist, male, aged 30, second year of training, work setting: psychiatric hospital

Mrs. M., a 42-year-old married woman, mother of three schoolchildren, had been admitted for treatment of depression after several months of unsuccessful psychiatric outpatient treatment. The consultant psychiatrist responsible for her requested that I see her for weekly psychotherapy sessions while in the hospital, and at the same time she was put on a new antidepressant. Mrs. M.'s childhood had been disrupted by WWII, as she had been one of those children that had been evacuated away from London to Cornwall, and she lost her father in the war. Her first marriage was not consummated, and she divorced her husband after one year. In her second and present marriage with a manager of a firm, serious relationship problems had developed, and she was afraid that this marriage, too, would end with a divorce. While in the hospital, she was not overtly depressed and even started a relationship with a male patient. Weekend leaves usually ended in disaster after being at home with her family. After six weeks the consultant decided to set a date of discharge so that she would have to face going home to her husband and children. He stopped her medication as he felt that this only added to her role of a helpless and ill patient. Her behavior soon became very difficult, and she started to act irrationally. She would rush into my room when I was seeing patients, begging and crying to be put back on medication because she felt worse and couldn't sleep any more. When I told the consultant, he refused to reconsider his decision and confirmed that she would be discharged on the set date. Two days before this date, early in the morning, she threw herself under a truck on the busy road passing the hospital.

D. The therapist: A psychiatrist, male, aged 42, 13 years of practice, work setting: private practice

Mr. J. was a creative and enterprising man who came from a very narrow-minded and pessimistic family background. He believed that he had successfully freed himself from his background. He was married and owned a clock repair service and was considered very reliable. He had never received any support from his parents. At the age of 48 he suddenly developed a severe depression which was resistant to the usual psychiatric treatment. He believed the onset of his depression was the deterioration of his eyesight (as had happened with his father) and his inability to do his work. It was as if he accused God for this misfortune. In spite of high doses of antidepressants and electro-convulsive therapy, his condition did not improve. When I saw him in my practice, his illness had already lasted for several years. He felt extremely bitter about psychiatrists and hospitals. The last admission had been against his will, taken from a family therapy session as he had said that he thought of killing himself. It was clear that he had a strong need for autonomy, yet in his helpless state he rejected everybody, including his wife and his daughters. He totally turned against his family and resisted all their attempts to help him. He would not accept more than a minimal medication from me and often brought back the tablets after having read everything available about possible side effects. He was in a constant fight against the world and himself, and for months he was in an awful state of agitated depression. He talked about suicide again and again. He wanted me to tell him how he could kill himself and to prescribe the necessary drugs. I replied that it was not my job and that I still believed that the depression could be lifted if we could establish an adequate antidepressant medication. I didn't understand why he continued to come to see me yet did not accept the help I offered. When I asked him he said: "You are the only person left in my life to whom I can talk." We talked about the good times in his past life and about his ideals and plans he had had. His condition got worse and worse. At home he stayed in his room and did not leave it even when his daughter and grandchild came for a visit. I had discussed the situation several times with his wife and both daughters, and everybody agreed that the worst thing that could happen to him would be to get him admitted to inpatient care against his will a second time. His daughter said that he had been an excellent father and she could not understand why he had changed so dramatically. He continued to come to see me altogether for over a year until one morning he drove into the forest and gassed himself with the car exhaust.

THERAPIST'S REACTIONS AFTER EXPERIENCING BOTH SUICIDES

The Female Therapist's Perspective

Both suicides were quite (even though at some level one knows it might happen but hopes that it just never will) a shock for me. There was a major difference between the two: for the first one, for Jane, I was the only one responsible, I was not experienced and almost convinced that this wouldn't happen had the therapist been more knowledgeable, more experienced and skillful. I was only two years older than my patient, so I developed a lot of doubts about my own competence as a therapist. Questions started to eat me up, some of them rational and constructive, some totally irrational and difficult to comprehend: What did I do wrong? What did I miss in the evaluation of her mental state? Why didn't I retreat from therapy before? Why did she do this to me? Was this a revenge of some sort? Is this because I am not a good enough therapist? Or maybe I am not a good person? Is this some sort of a punishment for something? I am probably no good for this vocation. Who will trust me now?

Will I trust myself? Is Jane's husband going to accuse me of killing her? What do my colleagues think of me now? Why did she do this when everything looked so promising? What a waste! She was not supposed to leave me like this. What do my superiors think of my work? I am so ashamed of my failure that I might even take my leave and disappear for a while.

After feelings of professional failure and incompetence, a very personal re-action hit me: I became sad and dysphoric, thought of Jane a lot, remembered her words that seemed now significant and perhaps might have been recog-nized before as desperate cries for help which I missed. The flashbacks of her usual, repetitive gestures came suddenly into me like a most painful blow. I felt as if I had lost a friend. There was no professional distance in my mind to this event. I even cried. I also told my husband about it, all in tears, and he tried to comfort me.

My supervisor offered to go through all the notes of our sessions, but I post-poned it for an indefinite time. The fear that my mistakes would be confirmed was too strong. I have never gotten myself to do it. I guess I was too frightened to find professional mistakes that were made in the course of therapy.

The case of Andrea was slightly different: Even though I regretted her sui-cide immensely, I managed to restore some professional distance, used some crisis intervention skills on myself and tried to talk with different colleagues as much as possible. From my clinical work with suicide survivors relatives and friends of the deceased, I knew that I had to work through my own grief as well as help the parents and my co-therapist. I called the parents and invited them to talk about Andrea and her reasons for the suicide. They came twice and a lot of things that were spoken then have helped not only them, but me as well. This time I went through my notes and talked to a family therapy team a lot--not only about the therapy performed, but about myself and my worries and sec-ond thoughts connected to Andrea's sudden decision to kill herself. In the end I understood more and accepted her will a bit easier.

The Male Therapist's Perspective

The first suicide in my second year of training was a blow that hit me totally unprepared. When I arrived at the hospital the patient's body had been taken away by the ambulance people, and the head nurse asked if I would inform her husband. My mind went blank. I was unable to do so. I was so shocked that I couldn't think clearly and didn't feel I could speak with family. I felt that I failed in my role as a doctor when I asked the head nurse to take over. The con-sultant psychiatrist, a normally soft and caring man, later that morning wanted to know what had happened, looked hurt and walked away. The case was never mentioned again. There was no team supervision, no case review, no de-briefing. I don't even know if the consultant ever spoke to the patient's hus-band. I reevaluated the case with my psychotherapy supervisor, but he did not follow up with me about the case. A few days after the suicide I developed a paranoid fear of her husband whom I had seen once with the patient. The thoughts that one day he would turn up and assault me or even kill me became more and more intrusive. I developed a fear of the dark: At night I got frightened to leave the house, especially when I had to go to the hospital when on duty. I never mentioned these fears to anyone, not even to my wife. I would have been ashamed to admit such irrational thoughts.

At that time there were several suicides per year in that small psychiatric hospital. In a way, what I learned as a young trainee in psychiatry was that suicide must be part of psychiatric routine and that, as in any accident/emergency unit, medical staff were simply expected to be strong enough to deal with this on their own. Maybe not surprisingly, two years later I started my first research project on suicide risk factors.

Twelve years later, the suicide of Mr. J. was a very different matter for me. I was sad and very touched when his wife called me during my practice hours to inform me of his death. Because of a teaching commitment I was unable to attend the funeral which I deeply regretted, as it would have meant a lot to the family and to me as well. I felt I had accompanied this man right into his death, and his unfortunate life story had touched me. I had admired him for what he had made out of his life, but his depression was like some malignant disease for which there appeared to be no cure. He was like Icarus who had lost his wings and saw no chance to ever fly again. I felt sympathy for this man and would have wanted to help him. But he didn't let me. I was slightly angry with him that he had killed himself without even bothering to leave a message for me. But then I told myself that he had had such a negative attitude towards the world around him that even I had been unable to give him a lifeline he could accept. Later, looking through the case notes I found a sentence he had copied from a book: "Hell: You sit here totally left by God and you feel that you cannot love any more, never again, and that you'll never meet another person again, never in eternity." His wife came to see me afterwards. She told me again that their marriage had been ideal for nearly 30 years and that he had been a good husband. She felt it had been right to let him go. So did I. I felt that the illness had been stronger than the patient, his family and myself. But doubts still crept into my mind. Had I really done everything for this man? Should I have seen him more frequently? Had I resigned too early? Working in a busy practice on my own I never had the opportunity to share my feelings with anyone. I still feel that I have to be able to cope with such events on my own.

DISCUSSION

Male therapist: So we both reacted strongly to the first suicide of a patient of ours, and we both didn't talk to a supervisor about the loss and all these strong emotions that came with it. It is well-known that therapists in their training years quite often encounter such an event and that they often feel left alone (Farberow, 2001, Grad, 1996). However, we both could have chosen to talk to someone, but we didn't. Why do you think we didn't choose to talk?

Female therapist: For me it was a matter of extreme feelings that my professional competence was questionable, resulting in suppression, guilt and shame, all of which I was very reluctant to share even with my supervisor. I would have had to have been approached by my supervisor and the appointment scheduled, even without my consent. However, I was able to speak about the incident with my closest people, mostly family and colleagues, which made it clear to me that I would need some support with my emotional reactions. Later I started to work with suicide survivors and did some research with therapists as suicide survivors.

M: Would you say that there is the difference between a male therapist and a female therapist?

F: Well, some data show (Grad et al., 1997) that women are more open to recognize and talk about feelings of guilt, shame, doubts they have about their professional knowledge, the need that they have to be comforted and so forth. Men tend to work more, but a lot of them talk to colleagues as well. I know that it helped me to talk, at least the second time. The first time, when I was blocked by my own feelings, it was more difficult to open up–maybe I had reacted more by the male stereotyped behavior.

M: But then, I think I may have a different attitude towards the death of a patient because early in my work as a doctor I was confronted with death. Amazingly, however, this never was a topic to be discussed (Michel, 1997, Fleming, 1997). Recently, I spoke to a general practitioner who told me that he had been called by a mother to confirm the death of her 35-year-old son after he had shot a bullet through his head. I asked him: How do you cope with this? He answered: "In my first years in practice it happened quite often and I got scared of being on call. But then I got used to it. I just continue to work. Sometimes, however, I wonder what it does to my system."

F: It might be true to a certain extent that the vocation makes a difference, but still, when I asked medical students about their need to be prepared for the suicide of their patient, and for death in general, most of them answered in a questionnaire that they have not enough knowledge and preparation on the topic whatsoever and they were extremely open to learn about it (Grad, 2000). When the (already practicing) physicians were asked the same question, they had a feeling they should have been able to cope with it by themselves, and they were not prepared to share their feelings with the others, especially not with their boss (Grad & Zavasnik, 1998). So obviously some defense mechanisms in connection with their role models play a part as well.

M: Do you think your reactions or coping mechanisms change with more years of experience? Maybe it is not only a matter of getting used to it, but also of feeling more competent in one's work. Maybe if it still happens, it is easier to say to yourself that you had done all that can reasonably be expected to do.

F: My hypothesis is that the suicide of a patient, when a therapist was fully engaged in a longer psychotherapy with the patient, inevitably triggers some emotional process in the therapist. The reactions and the coping skills of the therapist might be handled differently, depending on their experience, self-confidence, status, etc., but some inner turmoil (or at least questions, doubts, uneasiness) always exists. I don't imply that everybody should react in the same manner or that everybody needs the same procedure, but I am convinced that denial, suppression, ignoring or overlooking the event is not helpful (for anyone–young or old, man or woman, experienced or inexperienced!).

M: Much may be a question of attitudes: As a therapist do you see yourself as responsible for the cure or the well-being of the patient? Or how much free will do you attribute to the client/patient?

F: I do not believe that we can be responsible for the decisions about life and death of another person. We are responsible to talk to her/him continuously about the problems that lead to the decision and to be very professional and knowledgeable in the process. If we feel ourselves not competent enough, we should not only refer but accompany the person to another clinician who is more able to deal with the problems. Ultimately it is the choice of the client.

M: I believe we agree that each case of a suicide of a patient must be reviewed. Also, it is important that the therapist concerned chooses the person with whom he or she wants to talk it over.

F: What would be your message for the readers of this article?

M: You know, especially when I talk about the first suicide I still feel anger after all these years–anger with the consultant, who never ever spoke to me about the case or asked me how I felt. I know that he, too, probably felt helpless, but it is not really an excuse for a supervisor. So my main message is: Trainees must know that it is absolutely necessary to discuss the case with some senior person, and senior professionals must know that in an institution an atmosphere must be created where there is room and trust to talk about such sensitive matters. It is not heroic to be tough and deny the impact of a suicide on health professionals.

F: My true belief is that there are no rules on how to ease the pain and disappointment which a therapist feels after a patient commits suicide. The only rule is: Do not pretend it hasn't had an effect on you. Each therapist should follow his/her own direction about what to do and how to deal with her or his own reactions.

REFERENCES

Alexander D.A., Klein S., Gray N.M. and Eagles J.M. (2000) Suicide by patients: Questionnaire study of its effect on consultant psychiatrists. *BMJ*, 320,1571-4.

Brown, H. (1987). The impact of suicide on therapists in training. *Comprehensive Psychiatry*, 28, 101-112.

Brown H.N. (1987). Patient suicide during residency training: Incidence, implications and program response. *J Psych Educ*, 11/4, 201-216.

Farberow N.L. (2001). The therapist-clinician as survivor. In: *Suicide Risk and Protective Factors in the New Millennium* (Ed.), Grad O.T. Ljubljana, 11-21.

Fleming G. (1997). The isolated medical practitioner. *Crisis*, 18, 132-133.

Grad O.T. (1996). Suicide–How to survive as a survivor. *Crisis*, 17/3, 136-142.

Grad, O.T., Zavasnik, A. and Groleger, U. (1997). Suicide of a patient: Gender differences in bereavement reactions of therapists. *Suicide and Life-Threatening Behavior*. 27(4), 379-386.

Grad O.T. and Zavasnik A. (1998). The caregivers reactions after suicide of a patient. V: Kosky R.J. et al. (Eds.). *Suicide Prevention–The Global Context*. New York & London, Plenum Press. 287-291.

Grad O.T. (2000). A questionnaire applied to the students of Medical School in Ljubljana, Slovenia–not published, personal.

Grad O.T. and Michel K. (1994). Losing a patient by suicide: A male-female perspective. Fourth International Conference on Grief and Bereavement in Contemporary Society. Stockholm: 136.

Michel K. (1997). After suicide: Who counsels the therapist? *Crisis*, 18, 128-130.

Valente S.M. (1994). Psychotherapists reactions to the suicide of a patient. *American Journal of Orthopsychiatry*, 64, 614-621.

Touching the Heart and Soul of Therapy: Surviving Client Suicide

Pam Rycroft

SUMMARY. This is an account of the suicide of a young woman who had been raped at the age of thirteen, by five boys. Personal and professional implications will be discussed, including the experience of grief and trauma, the impact on work life and confidence, and the challenge to one's values and beliefs. The need for information about and support through legal processes will be explored. The medico-legal assumption that life is to be protected at all costs is examined. The importance for all to identify, understand and review our deepest values about life and death with clients and colleagues is asserted. *[Article copies available for a fee from The Haworth Document Delivery Service: 1-800-HAWORTH. E-mail address: <docdelivery@haworthpress.com> Website: <http://www.HaworthPress.com> © 2005 by The Haworth Press, Inc. All rights reserved.]*

KEYWORDS. Suicide, grief, suicide-professional impact

INTRODUCTION

Emma was 16, the same age as my daughter, when she came to my office that April day. She had come to meet another young sexual abuse survivor

Pam Rycroft is a psychologist who has worked in public psychiatry, community mental health, and at The Bouverie Centre, Victoria's Family Institute, where she has practised and taught family therapy for the last 16 years.

Address correspondence to: Pam Rycroft, The Bouverie Centre, 50 Flemington Street, Flemington, Victoria, Australia, 3031 (E-mail: p.rycroft@latrobe.edu.au).

[Haworth co-indexing entry note]: "Touching the Heart and Soul of Therapy: Surviving Client Suicide." Rycroft, Pam. Co-published simultaneously in *Women & Therapy* (The Haworth Press, Inc.) Vol. 28, No. 1, 2005, pp. 83-94; and: *Therapeutic and Legal Issues for Therapists Who Have Survived a Client Suicide: Breaking the Silence* (ed: Kayla Miriyam Weiner) The Haworth Press, Inc., 2005, pp. 83-94. Single or multiple copies of this article are available for a fee from The Haworth Document Delivery Service [1-800-HAWORTH, 9:00 a.m. - 5:00 p.m. (EST). E-mail address: docdelivery@haworthpress.com].

Digital Object Identifier: 10.1300/J015v28n01_07

who was to talk to her about possible membership in a group we were running for young sexual assault survivors. Emma had not had a positive experience of therapy: It seemed to re-traumatise her. It felt like a minor 'breakthrough' that she would consider this group. The meeting went well and Emma agreed to attend the next group session.

After a shaky start in therapy, work with her finally felt to be getting somewhere. Initially family sessions had been like walking on cut glass. Emma had not been able to tolerate the word "rape" being spoken; she would rush out of the room, distressed and angry. So much was unspeakable. Over time, she let me negotiate with her ways in which we could both talk about what needed to be said, including her right to let us know when it became too much to bear. On this occasion, she had been doing some heartwarming reminiscing with her parents. We had talked about the years before the trauma, as well as the time immediately afterwards, when she kept the 'voices' (reiterating the threats made by her perpetrators), and her other symptoms to herself. During this time her parents had been struggling to make sense of why their beautiful, talented daughter had suddenly become a rebellious, uncontainable, risk-taking 13-year-old. Family relationships, which had been strained to breaking point, seemed to be tolerating our touching some emotional wounds, albeit very gently. What was more, some were just beginning to show signs of some healing. That tenuous hold on hope against the pull of despair momentarily felt more robust.

When her mother arrived for a session without her father and Emma heard that he had walked out of home unexpectedly, her mood deteriorated steadily and significantly. Her mother wanted some time alone with the therapists to explain what had happened. By the time Emma joined us she was distracted, unavailable and appeared to be hearing the voices again. The most immediate need was to return her to her supervised accommodation, where she could be safe and supported. She had asked previously if I could see her for individual counseling, as well as continuing co-therapy with the family. This was a little outside of the mandate of our public family therapy center, but the director had agreed and I offered her an appointment early the next day. Her mother did not feel safe enough to drive her back alone, especially since Emma was insistent on meeting her friend at a suburban railway station, and neither I nor her mother felt she was safe to do this. It was late in the day and my co-therapist had to go onto a teaching program in the same building.

What followed was an attempt to act on a previously negotiated safety plan, which meant contacting a Protective Services worker, who, it was hoped, would arrange for Emma to be taken to secure and supported accommodation for the night. Emma, her mother and I sat in my office, with phone calls going to and fro, for more than an hour. Her mood ranged from calm and reflective to highly agitated: She took a number of cigarette breaks, first with her mother, then alone, while we were both on the phone. It was during one of these that she didn't come back into the room, and we realized that she had left the center. This seemed like previous times, and we assumed she had done what she used to do and made her own way across town to meet her friend, which she had seemed determined to do. After a fruitless search, and informing the police, I spent a brief time with Emma's mother and we then left to go to our cars. When I was driving out of the center into the main road with Emma's mother in her car behind me, I heard the repetitive clanging of the railway crossing boom gates. They were obviously stuck. When I saw the flashing lights of the ambulance my heart began to thump, I felt a cold sickness and I knew immediately something I hadn't previously even considered: that Emma had put herself in front of a passing train.

How could I not have predicted this? How could I have let this happen? She was just in my room. Yes, she was suicidal, but she had been suicidal for a long time, and usually went out with friends, drank, took drugs, did anything to induce unconsciousness, her only refuge, after which she would be found, dried out and returned into safe accommodation. Yes, she had come close to death in the past, but she had never talked of or attempted putting herself on the railway line. And things had been looking so much more hopeful lately: Just hours earlier she had been more open and positive than I had heard before. . . . How could this be? How could I have let her slip away so easily. . . . How could I have let her die? How can I ever work with young people at risk again? . . . I couldn't be trusted to keep them safe!

Six years later, I still hate the clanging sound of the bells on railway crossing boom gates. I still ask myself the same questions. I have found answers to some and not to others. Emma will always be large in my memory. She challenged me in a way that no other client ever has . . . not just because of her fragile, hair-breadth hold on life, but because she challenged some of my deepest values—my belief in life at all costs, my relentless pursuit of hope.

I tried to deal with Emma's death by researching the literature and presenting papers about the impact of suicide on families only to realize that I was trying to heal myself and make sense of how I could continue to work as a therapist. Emma's parents, who could have blamed us but shared their grief with us instead, who could have given up but asked us to continue working with them to help them survive as a family, assisted me to see that I was going through my process in partnership with them. At first, this was difficult to acknowledge. How could I ever compare my feelings to those who had lost a vibrant, talented and loving sister and daughter? What right did I have to grieve when I had let them all down so badly? And how could I, an experienced professional, admit to such feelings of shame and vulnerability without betraying my profession or myself?

I found that once I was able to acknowledge some aspects of the impact on me personally and professionally, and to investigate instead of deny the acute pain associated with Emma's death, it was a difficult but rewarding process. Initially, I was somewhat dismayed to find only one piece of writing that helped me make sense of what was happening to me. I discovered a chapter by

Frank Jones (1987) by accident. What a relief to read someone else's experience, to read this author's description of the double impact of suicide, both personal and professional. I hung on every word. It was some time later that an astute colleague heard my agony behind a stumbling, awkward question at a conference when I attempted to raise this topic. Where others responded by talking about suicide prevention techniques, he quietly took me aside later, talked a little about his experience, and directed me to James Hillman's book *Suicide and the Soul* (1997).

Hillman challenges psychology to make the study of the soul one of its main tasks. To do this, he points out, psychology would need to confront and not avoid the topic of death. Yvonne Hunter (1994) had the courage to write about the need to address issues of the soul in family therapy. While this paper does not cover the issue of suicide directly, it came closer to my experience than much of the literature on suicide generally.

It is not in any statistics or demographics or suicide prevention strategies that comfort or deeper understanding is to be found following the completed suicide of a client. It is in making some meaning out of that individual's act in the context of their "soul history" (Hillman, 1997) as distinct from their case history. Soul eludes definition; for me it incorporates the depths and the heights of human emotion, but goes beyond emotionality to include the physical as well as conscious and unconscious experience. Hunter (1994) describes this as related to family therapy: "Dropping into and therefore acknowledging the actual pain and suffering that is brought to therapy can lead to experiences that have such depth they could more properly be described as spiritual, or at least transformational" (p. 82).

The suicide of a client represented my greatest professional fear. I wondered how other more experienced therapists dealt with this fear. They were silent, as I had remained silent in my fear, simply hoping it would never happen to me. Surely professionals must experience such things all the time across the world–why the apparent conspiracy of silence about the impact of client suicide? One of Emma's protective workers, a wonderful, conscientious and caring young woman, left social work completely after Emma's death. It strikes me that if one of the results of silence is the loss of good, sensitive workers for our vulnerable clients, this is too high a cost.

Since Emma's death, two other young people with whom I had worked have completed suicide. I was not nearly as directly involved with either, and the impact was different, but it did contribute to my feeling of 'toxicity.' Therapy of its very nature involves a privileged intimacy. The suicide of someone with whom we have shared such an intimacy is ". . . the most wrenching agony of therapeutic practice. . . . It goes to the heart of therapy. Since we are each in a silent therapy with ourselves, the issue of suicide reaches into the heart of each of us" (Hillman, 1997, p. 192). Suicide also presents a profound ethical, legal and spiritual challenge to us individually as well as to us as a community.

Ethical and legal frameworks go so far, but not far enough to guide us through the spiritual questions and dilemmas.

One agony for me surrounded the idea that because I had come close to understanding why Emma embraced death as an ally, somehow I had colluded with her suicide. In the excruciating revision of things done and said, or not done or said, the smallest moments can be seen as pivotal and causal. In one pivotal conversation some twelve months before she died, Emma talked about death as a promise, a release, and a welcome refuge from the inescapable torment of living. I had no answer to her embracing death as the only permanent place of peace. Nor was it raised as a position to be argued–she talked of how everyone tended to dismiss her view of death, and argue against it, which only served to silence her and confirm her own view. Any attempts of my own to argue on the side of life would have silenced her and sounded hollow in my own ears and more self-protective than I cared to admit. I have never been so humbled, nor so agonizingly in touch with human vulnerability and my own limitations.

The closer I came to a genuine understanding of and empathy for Emma's strong relationship with death, the more moved I became and the less confident about what I had to offer her. In not finding the right words to dissuade her from her view, was I in fact colluding with the idea of death as the only solution? Would it have made a difference if during this conversation I had taken a stronger stand against death as a solution? Did I respond to her quiet despair in such a way that I failed the side of life and hope?

It would seem to me that there is a professional void that we confront with the suicide of a client, which leaves us struggling to find equilibrium, a position, and some sense of meaning. When our professional community has no clear voice, we are forced to find personal resources and examine our own inner voice for answers. The realm of 'professional' enters into one's personal life as at no other time, through thoughts, dreams and feelings (which I sometimes refer to as "burn-in," as distinct from "burn-out"). And our personal vulnerabilities and resources cannot help but enter into our professional lives. The personal and the professional become deeply intertwined.

It took some time to 'own' my grief, my shattered confidence and my doubts. I found myself engaging in private rituals (listening to Emma's favorite music; reading her poems over and over) and feeling embarrassed to speak of my powerful dreams. I dreaded colleagues being too quick to reassure me about my competence, and yet I needed their reassurance desperately. I wanted people not to dismiss my guilt but to help me examine the parameters of my responsibility, as well as what I might have done differently; to help me distinguish what was only apparent through hindsight.

SAFETY

I felt I had been working in a naïve, protected corner of my profession and the work so far had been a sort of 'sham.' Maybe other professionals had been through this many times, knew what to do, or wouldn't have let it happen in the first place, and I had just been operating with a deluded sense of 'this couldn't happen to me.' Yet I had often contemplated a client's suicide. I had lived through dreams and anxious Monday mornings wondering whether I would come to work to news of a client's death. Somehow I had escaped the reality until this time. I thought about the times that I had talked with clients about suicide, about how easy it was to hold the belief that clients who threatened suicide were only "calling for help." They didn't "really" want to die; they simply needed to let us know that they were struggling to find a reason to live.

The fact that a client could complete suicide meant that the world had changed, nothing was predictable any more, and it was no longer safe to assume anything. That a professional experience could be so overwhelming and challenging, and the fact that there seemed to be so few 'anchors' meant that just being at work felt unsafe for a little while. Finding avenues for expression of these early fears and feelings was crucial. It was not easy to express these at work: It takes "an enormous amount of courage to speak from the position of one's least empowered self" (Epstein, 2001).

Inspired by Jones (1987), I used my own family therapy network to advertise and begin a group for therapists who were survivors of client suicide (Victorian Association of Family Therapists' Inc. S.O.S. group). This was an open, self-help group, which became a strong source of support and action. It was the one place where it felt safe to say exactly whatever we felt without fear of judgment.

CONFIDENCE

Despite all the support and reassurance offered by colleagues, nothing was able to convince me that I hadn't failed professionally in the most public and extreme way possible, particularly given that I was the last professional to see Emma alive. Over time, I have come to accept that, with hindsight, there were things that I could have done differently that may have meant her surviving that night. But whether that meant she may have survived the next night, or the next, or the following years, I will never know.

I have learned that it is possible to build confidence again as a therapist, as long as there is sufficient support and backup over time. A very important part of this support is the acknowledgment that such an impact on confidence is a normal reaction to such an experience, rather than some pretence that one should be able to simply continue as before. I feel very much for young, less experienced workers who haven't had the chance to build the experience to know that we all have a mix of outcomes in our work. Those young people I had worked with whose will to live had survived their will to die were important to keep in mind at those times when my self-questioning became agonising.

Following the suicide of a client, the therapist needs a 'mentor,' someone who will help to make those decisions about how quickly to return to the normal work patterns and how quickly to return to working with people at risk. I imagine that this is a very individual decision; for my own part, one of the best and worst things that happened was that the day following Emma's suicide, I had a crisis call from another young client who was feeling actively suicidal. I could feel my own tendency to overreact, and felt that I was the wrong one to handle this. My director encouraged me to do what I felt I could and supported me by speaking to the young client himself, and sharing the decisions and the responsibility. As time has passed, I remain conscious of a sensitisation to suicidality and a tendency to want to protect myself against the experience. I don't believe that this is necessarily a bad thing, but I do believe it is important to be aware of the impact of our experience on our responses to clients, and to seek supervision and support professionally.

THE CHALLENGE TO BELIEFS

There are a number of professional beliefs that we hold; some conscious and acknowledged; some less so. Colin Murray-Parkes (1993) writes of the "assumptive world"–the human tendency to assume certain things, for example, that our children will outlive us; or that if we take reasonable precautions the world is a safe place. Whether it is at the level of family, local or international community (when a child dies or when events occur such as aeroplanes being used as weapons of mass destruction), our assumptive world is shattered.

A client suicide can no longer be assumed to be something that only happens to others. The fact that it can happen once means that it can happen again. Perceptions and judgments are called into question and this readily generalises to perceptions and judgments about other things in life. At the time of Emma's death I became acutely aware of some of my own naïve and self-aggrandising assumptions that were now untenable: that if I cared about my clients enough, they would be safe; that everyone can be helped by the right sort of help; that if I ask the right questions or say the right things, that will keep clients safe. One of the most challenging aspects of my work as a family therapist is to confront my own limitations. The purest of motivations, the hardest of work, and the highest of commitments sometimes is still not enough. We know this logically, but at the time of a client suicide, it smacks us across the face.

PROFESSIONAL IDENTITY CRISIS

I often work with students helping them to identify their core professional values and motivations or "telos" (Luepnitz, 1988). Within the helping professions, working toward decreasing distress and symptomatology is core to one's identity. Just as one aspect of a family's core identity is physical safety, with therapists one might expect emotional protection and safety. Suicide challenges the very nature of the family, and therapy. As Colin Murray-Parkes puts it (in Wertheimer, 1991), suicide is a rejection of the central supportive function, and faith in the family as a source of love and security is called into doubt.

Similarly, I believe, suicide can be felt to represent the most abject failure of the basic nature of therapy, at the highest possible cost. We ask ourselves: "What does it mean that a therapist cannot keep a client safe from the will to die?" "What sort of a therapist am I?" "Am I 'toxic'?" I used to think "Don't let me near any people at risk: They won't be safe with me." Post-suicide, families not only feel different, but bad, and this is often reinforced by community attitudes. Studies (e.g., Rudestam, 1987) have shown these families to be seen as blameworthy and less likeable. Therapists fear similar judgment by the professional community. This can be communicated in subtle and not so subtle ways. The day following Emma's death, the supervisor of her protective worker joined us on a phone conference line and asked me at one point: "Did you not think that the risk was serious enough to call the police directly?" In fact, we had been following the agreed safety plan in contacting Protective Services, but this question brought with it a strong message of criticism and blame to my ears at that particular time.

One of the most helpful things to me was hearing some of Emma's other treating professionals talk about their own fears that she could have suicided while in their care. One young worker talked about the many times Emma had run away from her, and her own dilemma mirroring mine, about how much to pursue and restrain and how much to let her go. An eminent psychiatrist after hearing my account of my last contact with Emma made the comment: "I just thought–there but for the Grace of God go I!" I could have hugged him. Hearing others' own personal feelings, particularly when they spoke from their own most vulnerable part, was one of the most helpful things for my healing.

Perspective takes some time to achieve, and attempts by others to reason with us in the immediate phase of shock will probably be futile. My experience tells me that time, talking with other therapists who have experienced client suicide, and permission to 'protect oneself' by working with professional support and backup are the factors that ultimately make it possible to regain a sense of identity as a good (but not perfect) therapist. It remains an issue to be watched. When I am working with young people at risk, I sometimes become aware of a strong 'pull' or bias that errs on the side of extreme conservatism in their treatment. I have to examine what my feelings are telling me, and whom I am trying to protect. It is useful to have a colleague to talk with, especially one who knows my work. Over time, it becomes possible to notice that other clients have, in fact, survived and done well after periods of suicidality. This can add to the poignancy and the sadness about the client who completed suicide, and more unanswerable questions about what may have happened had she or he survived that attempt. My experience also tells me that nothing builds confidence like success, and good work with our other clients is the best rehabilitation for therapists.

TRAUMA

Our colleagues should not become our therapists, but they can play a significant role in supporting us through such times. If the workplace does not allow for the expression of grief and trauma reactions, then there is a strong risk that such grief becomes "disenfranchised" (Doka, 1988), leading to more complex and difficult processes. This is not to say that simply suggesting time off from work is an appropriate response. For some this may be useful; others will feel it essential to continue working. What is important is having someone with whom to negotiate how to manage the therapist's own needs.

It is really important for the professional to be reminded that to experience some post-trauma symptoms is a sign of humanity and not weakness. Suicides can and do affect us physically, emotionally, and spiritually. They are never forgotten; however, like other major life events, the impact runs a course that can also lead to new understandings and growth, professionally and personally.

PERSONAL AND PROFESSIONAL BOUNDARIES

Professional codes of ethics also fall short of providing real guidance in response to questions such as: Should the helper have contact with the family, or further, see the family in therapy? Should I visit the grave–go to the funeral? Is it for me the person or the professional that I want to do this? Can they be distinguished at a time like this? If it is my own personal need, does this make it wrong? A colleague who shared her experience in a small self-help group for therapists surviving client suicide talked of her difficulty in sorting out which emotional issues were her own and how much emotional 'unfinished business' she had 'taken on' from her client. Most members of this small group described difficulty in the professional workplace with unspoken criticism in relation to any public expression of grief for the client. One was told outright that this was self-indulgent; another was said to be 'over-involved' with her client; another that it was simply explained by counter-transference. It seems that in many professional contexts grieving for clients is not sanctioned. Most of us had experienced some form of 'debriefing.' For me, that process felt more like a process of accountability. The others in the group also commented on the way that debriefing can be too easily and uncritically be seen as the single process whereby the workplace discharges its responsibility to the worker. More than one group member commented that the debriefing process felt more "real" with family members of the client than with colleagues. This pays tribute to the fact that an experience like this is primarily an intensely personal experience: As with any grief or trauma we gain most comfort and meaning with those who come closest to the experience. We need to trust our whole person to those with whom we share the experience, but we also need our colleagues to help us find meaning professionally. The personal becomes the professional, and the professional personal.

In this case, the fact that I was with Emma's mother at the scene of her death led to a particular impact. Going with her to identify the body, staying with Emma's parents through the early hours of the morning, all led to a particular poignant intimacy. Such experiences can't help but change the 'rules' for therapist-client relationships. But it didn't mean that we couldn't resume a working relationship. My co-therapist and I agreed to see Emma's parents for couple counselling following Emma's death: We did this because they asked us, but we didn't make the decision easily. In fact, it was my co-therapist who stopped in the middle of one of the early sessions and reflected on the possible impact of their daughter's suicide on their marriage. He had the courage to show his own feelings which enabled us all to cry together, not loudly, but gently, interspersed with laughter, and to 'speak the unspeakable.' This was a therapeutic intervention for both the couple and the therapists. It has given me faith in the importance of being 'real' in therapy, of having courage to use oneself and one's own vulnerabilities. I worried about the possibility that this contact may be as much for our own benefit and healing as for Emma's parents. We were conscious that our sense of responsibility and guilt could easily lead to a difficulty in making clinical decisions in any dispassionate way. We wondered whether we would be able to finish contact with the family. This led to agonizing doubts and self-questioning so that with every decision about whom to see and when, we asked ourselves, "For whose sake?" Finally, we decided to do something inspired by a much earlier conversation with Virginia Goldner (personal communication, 1993), which was to share our dilemma with the family. We talked about the experience and the work, and they helped us to be helpful in the way they needed. The couples work became a 'dance' which incorporated some very practical 'sorting out' of issues, as well as reflections on the impact, not only of Emma's suicide, but of the years leading up to it. When we relaxed and let the clients guide us in relation to what was helpful, we embarked on a constructive and useful therapeutic process which ended when they felt ready for it to end and left an 'open door' for any future issues.

CONCLUSION

Having had some fifteen years' professional experience without experiencing a client suicide contributed to a denial that it was ever likely to happen to me. And as long as I held to this belief, I failed to face my fear in any constructive way. The fact that it has happened, and that I have managed to continue working as a family therapist, gives me a sense of the strength which grows from feeling at my most vulnerable, and moving on from that feeling. I talk openly about the experience with colleagues and students in the hope that their own fears and experiences can be shared. It has helped me to be less afraid of other fears and to be more inclined to name them and seek help in tackling them.

Working with Emma's family after her suicide (against some professional opinion) showed me that rigidity should not govern clinical situations. I believe that if we come from a position of genuine trust and respect for our clients' opinions about what is in their own interest, they will let us know, and there is the potential for a truly mutually rewarding relationship. It was important to establish on what basis therapy might continue, and for all of us to 'keep each other on our toes' with regard to the agenda as well as when to finish. In the latter part of our contact with Emma's parents, we were able to reflect on the whole process of our contact, to talk about our initial difficulty in talking with them, and to learn from each other as clients and therapists.

Though painful, dealing with such a tragic situation and making sense of the experience leads to a sense of having 'moved through' a significant process which can't help but touch one's personal and professional life deeply. Indeed, it touches the heart and soul of therapy and life. As with any grief, it moves and changes over time, and can arouse a range of feelings, some agonising, some enriching. It was an experience of dread, and yet I have to acknowledge some sense of relief or comfort knowing it is possible to survive such feelings. I believe it is possible for an experience like this to enable us to sit more easily with clients' own strong feelings, without having to intervene to make ourselves feel better.

Professionally, the suicide of a client forces the therapist to face death as a reality, and we need to be mindful of the effect this may have on our practice. But it is possible that we can both respect this and not shy from it. I am now more likely, when it seems appropriate, to have conversations with clients about death and what it may represent to them. This does not make me an ally to suicide; rather, it brings the relationship with death "out of the closet" and open to examination and review.

Again, as with any grief, the survivor often looks at her or his own life through a different lens. One's priorities are suddenly up for review. When someone with whom we have had the privileged intimacy of a therapist-client relationship takes her or his own life, it leads to a lot of 'soul-searching,' not just about professional, but also about the deepest personal issues. It can get us in touch with what is important in our own lives and with what we have to be grateful for. It can also help to develop a new appreciation and commitment to our own personal relationships. Emma touched my soul deeply and continues to influence me.

REFERENCES

Doka, K.J. (1988). *Disenfranchised grief: Recognizing hidden sorrow*. Toronto: Lexington Books.

Epstein, M. (2001). The chocolate cake factor–'deep dialogue' in practice. Presentation at *Women Making Waves*. Women in Therapy conference. Lorne, Victoria.

Goldner, V. (1993). Personal communication.

Hillman, J. (1997). *Suicide and the soul*. (2nd Edition). Connecticut: Spring Publications.

Hunter, Y. (1994). Care of the soul in family therapy. *A.N.Z.J. Fam. Ther., Vol. 16, No. 2*. 81-87.

Jones, F.A. (1987). Therapists as survivors of client suicide. In E.J. Dunne, J.L. McIntosh and K. Dunne-Maxim (Eds.), *Suicide and its aftermath: Understanding and counseling the survivors* (pp. 126-141). New York: W.W. Norton & Company.

Luepnitz, D.A. (1988). *The family interpreted*. New York: Basic Books.

Parkes, C.M. (1993). Bereavement as a psychosocial transition: Processes of adaptation to change. In M.S. Stroebe, W. Stroebe & R.O. Hansson (Eds.), *Handbook of bereavement: Theory, research and intervention* (pp. 91-101). New York: Cambridge University Press.

Rudestam, K.E. (1987). Public perceptions of suicide survivors. In E.J. Dunne, J.L. McIntosh and K. Dunne-Maxim (Eds.), *Suicide and its aftermath*. New York: W.W. Norton.

Wertheimer, A. (1991). *A special scar: The experiences of people bereaved by suicide*. London: Routledge.

Suicide and the Law:
A Practical Overview
for Mental Health Professionals

Stephen R. Feldman
Staci H. Moritz
G. Andrew H. Benjamin

SUMMARY. The purpose of this chapter is to delineate how mental health professionals can prevent their clients from acting in a suicidal manner while protecting themselves against potential liability when a

Stephen R. Feldman, JD, PhD, is a licensed Washington State attorney and psychologist and has served on the faculties of local law and medical schools. He consults with both lawyers and mental health practitioners as part of his private practice. He is the author of several articles and one book published by American Psychological Association Press: *Law and Mental Health Professionals: Washington* (1998).

Staci H. Moritz is a law student at Seattle University School of Law, holds a Master of Arts in Clinical Psychology, and works as a social worker in mental health court for a Seattle public defender law firm.

G. Andrew H. Benjamin, JD, PhD, serves as Affiliate Professor of Law at the University of Washington. He has published 36 articles in psychology, law, and psychiatry journals and is the author of two books published by American Psychological Association Press: *Law and Mental Health Professionals: Washington* (1998) and *Family and Evaluation in Custody Litigation: Reducing Risks of Ethical Infractions and Malpractice* (2003).

Address correspondence to: Stephen R. Feldman, JD, PhD, 216 1st Avenue S., Suite 333, Seattle, WA 98121 (E-mail: Stephanjd@aol.com).

[Haworth co-indexing entry note]: "Suicide and the Law: A Practical Overview for Mental Health Professionals." Feldman, Stephen R., Staci H. Moritz, and G. Andrew H. Benjamin. Co-published simultaneously in *Women & Therapy* (The Haworth Press, Inc.) Vol. 28, No. 1, 2005, pp. 95-103; and: *Therapeutic and Legal Issues for Therapists Who Have Survived a Client Suicide: Breaking the Silence* (ed: Kayla Miriyam Weiner) The Haworth Press, Inc., 2005, pp. 95-103. Single or multiple copies of this article are available for a fee from The Haworth Document Delivery Service [1-800-HAWORTH, 9:00 a.m. - 5:00 p.m. (EST). E-mail address: docdelivery@haworthpress.com].

client attempts or completes suicide. In our increasingly litigious society mental health professionals can apply their understanding about the elements of legal liability in cases involving client suicidal behaviors to structure their services in a manner to meet their responsibility in treating potentially suicidal clients. *[Article copies available for a fee from The Haworth Document Delivery Service: 1-800-HAWORTH. E-mail address: <docdelivery@haworthpress.com> Website: <http://www.HaworthPress.com>*

KEYWORDS. Malpractice, negligence, breach of duty, confidentiality, lethality assessment, no-harm contracts

The most common form of legal action filed against clinicians is a suit alleging malpractice, which *Black's Law Dictionary* defines as ". . . failure to exercise the degree of care and skill that a (clinician) of the same (clinical) specialty would use under similar circumstances" (Garner, 1999). When legal action is brought against a clinician for malpractice, the legal theory is often one of negligence, a type of tort. A tort is a private or civil wrong resulting from a breach of legal duty owed by the defendant (e.g., the clinician) to the plaintiff (e.g., the client) which actually and proximately causes harm to the defendant (Garner, 1997). There are intentional torts, i.e., assault, battery, false imprisonment, etc., and there are unintentional torts, i.e., negligence. Most commonly, a client who brings a legal action against a clinician seeks to sue under a theory of negligence, which is a tort of omission: the failure of the clinician to have acted in accordance with reasonable skill and professional standards of care, and thereby to have caused harm to the plaintiff. In order for the court to find that the clinician was negligent in treating the client, the clinician must have reasonably foreseen the client's suicide and have failed to act appropriately, or the clinician must have acted unreasonably in evaluating or treating the client, thereby causing or resulting in the client's suicide (Kussman, 2000).

There are four basic elements of negligence: duty, breach, causation, and harm/damages. In a suit for malpractice, the specific form of negligence about which we are talking, the plaintiff must show that the clinician owed the client the duty of reasonable care; that the clinician breached that duty of care; that the breach of the duty actually and proximately (legally) caused the harm; and that measurable damages have resulted from the harm. The first element that must be proven in an action for malpractice against a clinician is that the clinician owed a duty of care to the client. It is widely recognized that a therapist bears a special relationship to a client that creates a duty of care based upon the clinician's presumed training and expertise in assessing the potential for suicide and the clinician's ability to take steps to prevent foreseeable suicide (*McLaughlin v. Sullivan*, 1983).

Therapists are routinely entrusted by their clients with sensitive and personal information with the expectation that the therapist will faithfully treat the client according to accepted professional standards of care. Among the duties clinicians owe their clients are duties of informed consent; confidentiality; thorough clinical assessment including assessment of suicide risk; and application of professional standards of care in preventing suicide if risk is identified (Packman & Harris, 1998). Collectively, these duties can be understood as fundamental elements of treating clients according to the professional standard of care, which is the standard that courts routinely apply when weighing whether or not a clinician has acted negligently. As will be seen below, in some instances, these duties can conflict.

In the event of legal action, after the plaintiff establishes that the clinician owes her or him a duty of care, the client will next have to prove that the clinician breached the duty of care. Breach of the duty of care under a theory of negligence involves failure of the clinician to act in accordance with established professional standards of care. Such breach may involve claims of breach of confidentiality; failure to properly assess or treat (foreseeability) that leads to a client's suicide attempt or completion; failure to warn family members or law enforcement about the client's suicidality if such a warning is permitted under the laws of the state regulating the mental health professional; or failure to confine a suicidal client appropriately if such confinement is mandated by the laws of the state. The clinician's faithful adherence to the professional standard of care and the laws of the clinician's state does not require that the clinician be clairvoyant in predicting clients' suicidality.

Prediction of suicidality tends to produce a high rate of false-positives (Packman & Harris, 1998). Sound clinical judgment, rather than unfailingly accurate prediction of suicidal behaviors, is fundamental to avoiding potential liability when treating suicidal or potentially suicidal clients. Courts are unlikely to assign error where a clinician has acted as a reasonable, similarly trained clinician would in properly assessing and planning the client's care (Packman & Harris, 1998). As long as the clinician provides reasonable evaluation and subsequent treatment, a clinician's mistaken judgment is insufficient to prove breach of duty.

Informed consent is one of the means by which the clinician discloses to the client the method of treatment, risks and potential outcomes, and policies regarding confidentiality and duties to expose confidences. Many jurisdictions call for the clinician to reveal client confidences whenever the client is mentally ill, rising to the level of psychotic behavior in most jurisdictions, and poses a danger to self either because of suicidality or grave disability (inability to take care of basic life needs to sustain survival). Many states have specific guidelines for when, if ever, a breach of confidentiality (warning others of the client's suicidality or evaluation for confinement) is required, and it is important that clinicians familiarize themselves with such laws in their jurisdictions. Some courts have held that clinicians owe no duty to report suicidality, citing potential erosion of confidentiality and thus the therapeutic alliance, as seen in one of the seminal cases on clinician liability, *Bellah v. Greenson* (1978). Such jurisdictions believe that prevention of such suicidal acts is more likely to occur if the client's confidences are more fully protected and the client's speaking out about their behavior is not chilled by incursions on confidentiality. However, other courts have held clinicians liable for failure to warn family members of clients of potential suicidality associated with certain medical or psychological conditions (*Wozniak v. Lipoff,* 1988; *Smith v. New York City Health & Hospitals Corp.,* 1995).

Often, an acceptable breach of the duty of confidentiality will occur when the clinician has good reason to believe that her client is at risk of self-harm or suicide. However, the best way to forestall potential liability resulting from a breach of confidentiality is for clinicians, during the informed consent process, to disclose to their clients the clinician's policies and governing laws that require breach of confidentiality ("mandatory reporting" in some states) that serve the interest of protecting the client's safety. It is good professional practice for clinicians to include this information in both the oral consent process and in the written disclosure statement that occurs and is provided to the client in the first visit. The client's informed consent to such disclosures and any discussion about potential disclosures is documented in the clinical record. With the advent of the federal Health Insurance Portability and Accounting Act (HIPAA) that contains privacy provisions that are in effect as of April 14, 2002, this documentation is required nationwide. Later, if suicidal ideation or behavior emerges, the clinician can discuss the informed consent process again as applied to the treatment and use such a discussion to deepen the therapeutic alliance by reminding the client of the limitations imposed upon the clinician by the law in revealing certain confidences. Planning about how to manage the suicidal ideation is then more likely to occur as a collaboration rather than an adversarial process.

When the imminence of suicidality becomes apparent, it is in both the clinician's and the client's best interest for the clinician to take the following steps in assessing and preventing lethality: Thoroughly assess the risk, including an assessment of motivation; determine specific plans and the means to carry out the plans; coordinate care among all relevant treatment providers and family members to the extent allowable in your jurisdiction; develop a safety plan with the client including emergency contact information; utilize emergency measures such as obtaining a evaluation of confinement necessity by the appropriate authorities; inventory and account for weapons or drugs in the client's possession; be mindful of destabilizing events and significant traumatic anniversaries that are upcoming; repeatedly assess lethality throughout the period of heightened risk; and finally, document all interventions in the clinical record (Benjamin & Feldman, 1998).

It is not wise to rely only on a "no-harm" contract. These are popular and often recommended. There is nothing wrong with such a written agreement, but standing alone, it will mean little clinically or legally. Such a contract must be seen as a part of a more complete intervention strategy and should be integrated into the therapeutic relationship. Most important is to assess repeatedly for lethality throughout the period of heightened risk and document all interventions in the clinical record.

When, if ever, is it permissible to release treatment records or information for a deceased client to a family member or other party? Although only two states (Washington and Montana) have to date adopted the Uniform Health Care Information Act that specifically describes person(s) authorized by law to act for the deceased (client), most states have similar laws that provide that any release of confidential treatment materials is only permissible when made to the decedent's legal representative, most commonly estate administrators or executors and legal guardians. For instance, in the state of Washington, in addition to the Uniform Health Care Information Act, there is a provision for the access to a decedent's records which is typical of most jurisdictions which states ". . . all information and records compiled, obtained, or maintained in the course of providing services to either voluntary or involuntary recipients of services at public or private agencies shall be confidential . . . [and] . . . may be disclosed only . . . To a patient's next of kin, guardian, or conservator, if any, in the event of death" (RCW 71.05.390).

One should be aware, however, that although a patient or her/his personal representative in the event of death (for any reason) has rights of access to records, there is also a provision for denial of access to those records if the clinician believes that such access would result in harm or injury to the patient, or a breach of the confidentiality of a third party who provided the information on the understanding of confidentiality. This is true under most state law and under the terms of the new HIPAA. Whether a personal representative legally stands in the shoes of the decedent for purposes of denial of access to records is a question that has not yet been tested in the courts.

In instances where clients or their families have sued clinicians following the client's suicide attempt or completion, the court will determine whether the plaintiff has standing (a legal standard that differs in the law of the various states but typically establishes who can file a malpractice suit, e.g., a wrongful death action, for the wrongful death of the client for the benefit of heirs and those who might have been dependent on the decedent client). The court will also determine, with respect to the alleged negligent act or acts whether the clinician acted in the way a reasonable clinician of equivalent training and credentials would have acted. The reasonableness of the clinician's actions, either affirmative or omissive, will be viewed in the light of the specific fact pattern and circumstances of each unique clinical case (Kussman, 2000).

One line of defense that clinicians may raise is that a patient assumed the risk in participating in therapy. However, such a defense has consistently been rejected because, the courts reason, a patient does not knowingly and voluntarily assume the risk that the clinician will treat the patient with anything less than the professional standard of care (Kussman, 2000). The risk of treating suicidal or potentially suicidal clients is borne primarily by the clinician, hence the necessity of adequate assessment, peer consultation, documentation, and affirmative measures to protect foreseeable suicidal clients. Although the risk is usually borne by the treating clinician, courts have, on occasion, found family members to be comparatively negligent, or partially negligent according to apportionment of the fault. If a clinician foresees that a client may be suicidal, makes appropriate recommendations to the client's family to ensure the client's safety, the family then fails to follow the clinician's advice, and the client completes suicide (*Paddock v. Chacko*, 1988), the family may be deemed partially responsible.

A clinician will not be held liable for negligence in failing to prevent suicide or a suicide attempt if the suicidality is not foreseeable (Kussman, 2000). Clinicians are not held liable for honest errors in judgment, provided that their evaluations and treatment of the client in the specific situation in question do not fall below the professional standard of care. If after a careful, documented risk assessment the clinician is reasonably unable to find indicators of suicidality, i.e., the client denying suicidal thoughts, wishes, plans, or a history of attempts, the clinician will not be held liable if the client completes suicide, having given no clear indication to the clinician of her or his intentions. However, if the plaintiff can show that the clinician's affirmative or omissive acts fall below the professional standard of care upheld by reasonable, similarly credentialed clinicians, liability will be imposed (*Edwards v. Tardiff*, 1977).

If a client indicates that suicidal ideation is present, the clinical record of such an assessment is made stronger if the clinician has engaged in paid professional consultation or peer consultation and the corroborating findings of the consultants are also noted in the record. Yet again, the burden rests on the clinician to assess with due diligence and to document the conversations with the client and consultant(s) about suicidal ideation or behaviors.

More than a general link between the clinician's alleged negligence and the client's suicide is necessary to find liability on the part of the clinician. After duty of care and breach of such duty is shown, the defendant must show that the clinician's negligence caused the client's suicide. In the law, there are two types of causation: actual and proximate. In order to show actual causation, the plaintiff must show that the clinician's negligent conduct actually caused the client's injuries (Henderson, Pearson & Siliciano, 1999). Actual causation can be thought of as "but for" causation: but for the clinician's omission, the harm would not have resulted to the client. Proximate cause is legal causation, i.e., suicide must have been foreseeable to the clinician. If the suicide was foreseeable but the clinician failed to intervene, the clinician's acts may be found to be the proximate cause of the client's suicide. A contemporaneous consultation that discussed all of the assessment factors and led to an agreement about a reasonable course of action in light of the assessment can effectively diminish a jury ever finding that the clinician was negligent. Both actual and proximate causation must be proven for a clinician to be found liable for negligence. In *Farwell v. Un*, 1990, a negligence action failed because of no proximate cause. A physician had been treating a depressed man with antidepressant medication for five months. The man told his wife that he had attempted suicide, of which the wife informed the doctor. The physician then recommended inpatient treatment beginning immediately, to which the man and his wife agreed. The following day the physician learned that the man had failed to admit himself to the hospital. The physician then spoke with the man's wife, who reported that the man was feeling better. The physician saw the man again seven days later following a referral from another psychiatrist the man had been seeing in the interim. In this meeting, the man again agreed to hospitalize himself. The following day the man completed suicide.

Although it may seem to a reasonable clinician that the physician should not have left admission to the hospital up to the client himself when such client was imminently suicidal, the court found the physician not liable for the man's suicide, reasoning that even if the physician's care before the first suicide attempt was negligent, the link between the negligent care and the man's suicide ten days later was too tenuous to show causation (*Farwell v. Un*, 1990).

In addition to showing that the clinician owed the client or plaintiff a duty of care that the clinician subsequently breached, as well as showing actual and proximate causation, a plaintiff must show that as a result of the clinician's affirmative or omissive acts, harm causing measurable damages resulted. Harm will likely be evident, provided that duty, breach, and causation are shown, when the client has either attempted or completed suicide. For instance, the estate of a decedent client may be able to recover for the pain and suffering of the decedent. This may be very little if it cannot be proven that the person suffered mental or physical pain between the wrongful act and the death. However, the beneficiaries of an estate might recover more if they can prove loss of economic benefit such as the support that the decedent was providing. If the decedent was supporting aging parents or minor children, the damages could be very substantial. However, if there was no one dependent, the likelihood of any legal action is quite diminished, although still possible in the form of loss of consortium claims, i.e., the loss of company, care and love of a spouse. Thus, in many suits for wrongful death, two different measures of damages might apply for the entities that are entitled to bring suit: the estate for pain and suffering to the decedent, and the beneficiaries for the economic loss to the dependents and the loss of consortium that the clinician may be considered to have caused.

Regardless of the clinical orientation of the clinician, the recommended protocol for assessing suicidality is rather standard. In the initial assessment, and periodically thereafter, as the client's behavior indicates the reemergence of suicidal ideation or planning, the clinician directly reassesses the client and records the findings of the assessment. The clinician evaluates the suicidal thoughts, plans, and attempts, as the client may not independently broach the subject out of shame, embarrassment, or fear (Morrison, 1995). The clinician's failure to inquire about suicidality, when clinical signs of suicidal ideation or behavior emerge, may prove lethal for the patient and may later give rise to legal action against the clinician for negligence in assessment and diagnosis. In the absence of evidence to the contrary, a clinician may safely accept a client's denial of suicidality when asked directly. However, if the clinician senses hesitation, ambivalence, or mood incongruity in the client's response, a more detailed inquiry is in order (Morrison, 1995).

A thorough understanding of the nature and gravity of any previous suicide attempts or active ideation will allow the clinician to anticipate possible recurring attempts and plan for the client's care in a clinically sound, liability reducing fashion. Such an understanding will help the clinician predict, based on clinical judgment, what the client may do next with respect to suicidality and what steps the clinician must take to ensure the patient's safety as much as possible (Morrison, 1995). In judging the seriousness of any prior suicide attempts, the clinician should ask about and record the level of physical harm in the prior attempt and assess how resolute the client is in a wish and intent to die (Morrison, 1995). A request for prior clinical records should be made and their review should occur as part of the lethality assessment. When the clinician is able to ascertain that the client is an imminent risk of harm, hospitalization should be carefully considered. When, however, the clinician perceives a risk, and according to sound clinical judgment, believes the risk can be best managed in the outpatient setting by means of the relationship between clinician and client, including a medication evaluation, risk is reassessed whenever suicidal ideation or behavior reemerges and acted upon according to accepted professional standards.

In summary, the best protection against liability for negligence resulting from a client's suicidality is to adhere to accepted standards of care of one's clinical profession in assessment, diagnosis, care planning and treatment; to familiarize oneself with jurisdictional guidelines addressing confidentiality and breach of confidentiality; to ensure that clinical interactions and clinical decisions are carefully documented in the client's permanent record; and to seek professional or peer consultation, particularly when inexperienced, uncomfortable or uncertain.

REFERENCES

Bellah v. Greenson, 146 Cal.Rptr. 535. Cal.App.,1978.

Benjamin, G.A.H., Rosenwald, L.A., & Feldman, S.R. (1998). *Law & mental health professionals: Washington.* Washington, D.C.: American Psychological Association Press.

Edwards v. Tardiff, 240 Conn. 610, 692 A.2d 1266. Conn.,1997.

Farwell v. Un, 902 F.2d 282. C.A.4 (Md.),1990.

Garner, B.A. (Ed.) (1999). *Black's law dictionary*. St. Paul, MN: West Group.

Henderson, J.A., Pearson, R.N., & Siliciano, J.A. The torts process. Gaithersburg, N.Y.: Aspen.

Kussman, P.C. (2000). Liability of doctor, psychiatrist, or psychologist for failure to take steps to prevent patient's suicide. In *American law reports 5th*. St. Paul, MN: West Group.

McLaughlin v. Sullivan, 461 A.2d 123 N.H.,1983.

Morrison, J. (1994). *The first interview*. New York, N.Y.: The Guilford Press.

Packman, W.L. & Harris, E.A. (1998). Legal issues and risk management in suicidal patients. In Bongar, B., Berman, A.L., Maris, R.W., Silverman, M.M., Harris, E.A., & Packman, W.L. (Eds.), *Risk management with suicidal patients* (pp. 150-186). New York. N.Y.: The Guilford Press.

Paddock v. Chacko, 522 So.2d 410. Fla.App. 5 Dist.,1988.

Revised Code of Washington, RCW 71.05.390.

Smith v. New York City Health and Hospitals Corp., 621 N.Y.S.2d 319. N.Y.A.D. 1 Dept.,1995.

Wozniak v. Lipoff. 750 P.2d 971 Kan.,1988.

Index

Faces of Women and Aging, edited by Nancy D. Davis, MD, Ellen Cole, PhD, and Esther D. Rothblum, PhD (Vol. 14, No. 1/2, 1993). *"This uplifting, helpful book is of great value not only for aging women, but also for women of all ages who are interested in taking active control of their own lives." (New Mature Woman)*

Refugee Women and Their Mental Health: Shattered Societies, Shattered Lives, edited by Ellen Cole, PhD, Oliva M. Espin, PhD, and Esther D. Rothblum, PhD (Vol. 13, No. 1/2/3, 1992). *"The ideas presented are rich and the perspectives varied, and the book is an important contribution to understanding refugee women in a global context." (Contemporary Psychology)*

Women, Girls and Psychotherapy: Reframing Resistance, edited by Carol Gilligan, PhD, Annie Rogers, PhD, and Deborah Tolman, EdD (Vol. 11, No. 3/4, 1991). *"Of use to educators, psychotherapists, and parents–in short, to any person who is directly involved with girls at adolescence." (Harvard Educational Review)*

Professional Training for Feminist Therapists: Personal Memoirs, edited by Esther D. Rothblum, PhD, and Ellen Cole, PhD (Vol. 11, No. 1, 1991). *"Exciting, interesting, and filled with the angst and the energies that directed these women to develop an entirely different approach to counseling." (Science Books & Films)*

Jewish Women in Therapy: Seen But Not Heard, edited by Rachel Josefowitz Siegel, MSW, and Ellen Cole, PhD (Vol. 10, No. 4, 1991). *"A varied collection of prose and poetry, first-person stories, and accessible theoretical pieces that can help Jews and non-Jews, women and men, therapists and patients, and general readers to grapple with questions of Jewish women's identities and diversity." (Canadian Psychology)*

Women's Mental Health in Africa, edited by Esther D. Rothblum, PhD, and Ellen Cole, PhD (Vol. 10, No. 3, 1990). *"A valuable contribution and will be of particular interest to scholars in women's studies, mental health, and cross-cultural psychology." (Contemporary Psychology)*

Motherhood: A Feminist Perspective, edited by Jane Price Knowles, MD, and Ellen Cole, PhD (Vol. 10, No. 1/2, 1990). *"Provides some enlightening perspectives. . . . It is worth the time of both male and female readers." (Contemporary Psychology)*

Diversity and Complexity in Feminist Therapy, edited by Laura Brown, PhD, ABPP, and Maria P. P. Root, PhD (Vol. 9, No. 1/2, 1990). *"A most convincing discussion and illustration of the importance of adopting a multicultural perspective for theory building in feminist therapy. . . . This book is a must for therapists and should be included on psychology of women syllabi." (Association for Women in Psychology Newsletter)*

Fat Oppression and Psychotherapy, edited by Laura S. Brown, PhD, and Esther D. Rothblum, PhD (Vol. 8, No. 3, 1990). *"Challenges many traditional beliefs about being fat . . . A refreshing new perspective for approaching and thinking about issues related to weight." (Association for Women in Psychology Newsletter)*

Lesbianism: Affirming Nontraditional Roles, edited by Esther D. Rothblum, PhD, and Ellen Cole, PhD (Vol. 8, No. 1/2, 1989). *"Touches on many of the most significant issues brought before therapists today." (Newsletter of the Association of Gay & Lesbian Psychiatrists)*

Women and Sex Therapy: Closing the Circle of Sexual Knowledge, edited by Ellen Cole, PhD, and Esther D. Rothblum, PhD (Vol. 7, No. 2/3, 1989). *"Adds immeasurably to the feminist therapy literature that dispels male paradigms of pathology with regard to women." (Journal of Sex Education & Therapy)*

The Politics of Race and Gender in Therapy, edited by Lenora Fulani, PhD (Vol. 6, No. 4, 1988). *Women of color examine newer therapies that encourage them to develop their historical identity.*

Treating Women's Fear of Failure, edited by Esther D. Rothblum, PhD, and Ellen Cole, PhD (Vol. 6, No. 3, 1988). *"Should be recommended reading for all mental health professionals, social workers, educators, and vocational counselors who work with women." (The Journal of Clinical Psychiatry)*

Women, Power, and Therapy: Issues for Women, edited by Marjorie Braude, MD (Vol. 6, No. 1/2, 1987). *"Raise[s] therapists' consciousness about the importance of considering gender-based power in therapy . . . welcome contribution." (Australian Journal of Psychology)*

Dynamics of Feminist Therapy, edited by Doris Howard (Vol. 5, No. 2/3, 1987). *"A comprehensive treatment of an important and vexing subject." (Australian Journal of Sex, Marriage and Family)*

A Woman's Recovery from the Trauma of War: Twelve Responses from Feminist Therapists and Activists, edited by Esther D. Rothblum, PhD, and Ellen Cole, PhD (Vol. 5, No. 1, 1986). *"A milestone. In it, twelve women pay very close attention to a woman who has been deeply wounded by war." (The World)*

Women and Mental Health: New Directions for Change, edited by Carol T. Mowbray, PhD, Susan Lanir, MA, and Marilyn Hulce, MSW, ACSW (Vol. 3, No. 3/4, 1985). *"The overview of sex differences in disorders is clear and sensitive, as is the review of sexual exploitation of clients by therapists. . . . Mandatory reading for all therapists who work with women." (British Journal of Medical Psychology and The British Psychological Society)*

Women Changing Therapy: New Assessments, Values, and Strategies in Feminist Therapy, edited by Joan Hamerman Robbins and Rachel Josefowitz Siegel, MSW (Vol. 2, No. 2/3, 1983). *"An excellent collection to use in teaching therapists that reflection and resolution in treatment do not simply lead to adaptation, but to an active inner process of judging." (News for Women in Psychiatry)*

Current Feminist Issues in Psychotherapy, edited by The New England Association for Women in Psychology (Vol. 1, No. 3, 1983). *Addresses depression, displaced homemakers, sibling incest, and body image from a feminist perspective.*

BOOK ORDER FORM!

Order a copy of this book with this form or online at:
http://www.haworthpress.com/store/product.asp?sku=5106

Therapeutic and Legal Issues for Therapists
Who Have Survived a Client Suicide
Breaking the Silence

____ in softbound at $19.95 (ISBN: 0-7890-2377-6)
____ in hardbound at $39.95 (ISBN: 0-7890-2376-8)

COST OF BOOKS _____

POSTAGE & HANDLING _____
US: $4.00 for first book & $1.50
for each additional book
Outside US: $5.00 for first book
& $2.00 for each additional book.

SUBTOTAL _____

In Canada: add 7% GST. _____

STATE TAX _____
CA, IL, IN, MN, NJ, NY, OH & SD residents
please add appropriate local sales tax.

FINAL TOTAL _____

If paying in Canadian funds, convert
using the current exchange rate.
UNESCO coupons welcome.

⊔ BILL ME LATER:
Bill-me option is good on US/Canada/
Mexico orders only; not good to jobbers,
wholesalers, or subscription agencies.

⊔ Signature _____

⊔ Payment Enclosed: $ _____

⊔ PLEASE CHARGE TO MY CREDIT CARD:
⊔ Visa ⊔ MasterCard ⊔ AmEx ⊔ Discover
⊔ Diner's Club ⊔ Eurocard ⊔ JCB

Account # _____

Exp Date _____

Signature _____
(Prices in US dollars and subject to change without notice.)

PLEASE PRINT ALL INFORMATION OR ATTACH YOUR BUSINESS CARD

Name	
Address	
City	State/Province	Zip/Postal Code
Country	
Tel	Fax
E-Mail	

May we use your e-mail address for confirmations and other types of information? ⊔ Yes ⊔ No We appreciate receiving
your e-mail address. Haworth would like to e-mail special discount offers to you as a preferred customer.
We will never share, rent, or exchange your e-mail address. We regard such actions as an invasion of your privacy.

Order From Your **Local Bookstore** or Directly From
The Haworth Press, Inc. 10 Alice Street, Binghamton, New York 13904-1580 • USA
Call Our toll-free number (1-800-429-6784) / Outside US/Canada: (607) 722-5857
Fax: 1-800-895-0582 / Outside US/Canada: (607) 771-0012
E-mail your order to us: orders@haworthpress.com

For orders outside US and Canada, you may wish to order through your local
sales representative, distributor, or bookseller.
For information, see http://haworthpress.com/distributors

(Discounts are available for individual orders in US and Canada only, not booksellers/distributors.)

Please photocopy this form for your personal use.
www.HaworthPress.com

BOF04

T - #0599 - 101024 - C0 - 212/152/7 - PB - 9780789023773 - Gloss Lamination